Learning
Psychiatry
through
MCQ

Learning Psychiatry through MCQ

A Comprehensive Text

Edited by

Tom Sensky

with contributions from Thomas R. E. Barnes, Steven R. Hirsch, Anthony G. Jolley, Peter F. Liddle, Eric Shur and Christopher Thompson

All members of the Department of Psychiatry, Charing Cross and Westminster Medical School, London, UK

A Wiley Medical Publication

JOHN WILEY & SONS
Chichester · New York · Brisbane · Toronto · Singapore

Library of Congress Cataloging-in-Publication Data:

Learning psychiatry through MCQ/edited by Tom Sensky; with
    contributions from Thomas R. E. Barnes . . . [et al.].
        p. cm.—(A Wiley medical publication)
    ISBN 0 471 91896 2 (pbk.)
    1. Psychiatry—Examinations, questions, etc.   I. Sensky, Tom.
II. Barnes, Thomas R. E.   III. Series.
    [DNLM: 1. Psychiatry—examination questions.   WM 18 L438]
    RC457.L43 1988
    616.89'0076—dc19
    DNLM/DLC
    for Library of Congress   88-223
                                                                      CIP

British Library Cataloguing in Publication Data:

Learning psychiatry through MCQ.
    1. Medicine. Psychiatry. Questions &
    answers
    I. Sensky, Tom   II. Barnes, Thomas R. E.
    III. Series
    616.89'0076

    ISBN 0 471 91896 2

Typeset by Acorn Bookwork, Salisbury, Wilts
Printed in Great Britain by Anchor Brendon Ltd., Tiptree, Essex

Contents

Foreword vii

Preface ix

1 Basic Concepts 1

2 Organic Disorders 21

3 Schizophrenia 47

4 Affective Disorders 67

5 Neuroses 87

6 Personality Disorders 103

7 Substance Abuse and Dependence 109

8 Eating Disorders 123

9 Suicide and Deliberate Self-harm 129

10 Sexual Function and its Abnormalities 135

11 Child Psychiatry and Mental Handicap 145

12 Psychiatry and Medicine 155

13 Treatments 179

14 Clinical Cases 205

Appendix 255

Subject Index 257

Foreword

Learning is always a challenge, but often the first challenge is to overcome a lack of interest and fascination because the student lacks an initial grasp of the subject. The traditional textbook sets out a standard descriptive account of the main conditions in psychiatry, their physical symptoms and signs, aetiology and treatment. However, students lacking experience of patients have difficulty discerning what are the most important features which distinguish one syndrome or diagnosis from another and what are the most important facts to be focused on. This book is set out to do just that—engage interest from the outset by identifying the key questions that need to be answered, posing them to the reader, and then answering them. It is meant to focus the student's attention on the most discerning issues and help him discriminate between the key facts and the less important ancillary ones. In this sense it fills a much needed gap in the information available to medical students and young doctors starting out to learn psychiatry. Educators are always quick to emphasise the importance of the problem-solving approach; this requires the student to reason with the facts, not just repeat them. The case histories section of this book provides an opportunity to exercise one's newly acquired clinical knowledge and apply it to a clinical problem as it would usually be approached under clinical conditions; the reader is taken through each stage of decision making from assessment and diagnosis to treatment, testing the student's grasp of facts in a clinical context and demonstrating the clinical relevance of basic facts.

This is the first such book written primarily for medical students, but it will be equally valuable for the young doctor starting to train in clinical psychiatry as a specialty.

The book came from a collaborative effort of the academic psychiatry staff of Charing Cross and Westminster Medical School, but was directed, shaped and honed by Dr Sensky who initiated the effort and nurtured it throughout. It reflects interest in trying to convey to students the most important issues of clinical knowledge, and Dr Sensky's success as a teacher in reviewing psychiatry with students just prior to their final examinations. We believe it will provide medical students and young doctors with a stimulating but helpful 'something extra' in their introduction to clinical psychiatry.

STEVEN R. HIRSCH

Preface

The idea for this book came originally from our students. Faced with multiple choice questions in many of their examinations, they asked for some sample questions in psychiatry geared to their particular needs. This book is, however, much more than simply a collection of multiple choice questions. The text is intended to provide the reader with a comprehensive account of general adult psychiatry, suitable for medical undergraduates.

No undergraduate textbook can be truly comprehensive. The contents of this book reflect the psychiatry teaching at our own medical school. There is emphasis on major psychiatric illness but we have also paid attention to the integration of psychiatry into clinical practice, covering aspects of psychiatry commonly encountered in primary care and in the general hospital. However, the reader is expected to acquire from elsewhere further knowledge about some topics, notably child psychiatry and mental handicap. We have made a particular effort to cover management of psychiatric problems, embracing psychological and social as well as physical approaches. This is especially important in the final section of the book, in which we have sought to integrate basic information in a clinically relevant manner centred on individual case histories.

The book is divided into sections or chapters, resembling those found in most conventional psychiatry textbooks. Within a section, each question and its accompanying text cover a circumscribed topic. This format has, to some extent, determined the way in which information is presented in the book. Different aspects of a particular topic may be covered in more than one question. To assist the reader using the book as a textbook or a source of reference, the symbol ★ in the text identifies indexed topics on which further information can be found elsewhere in the book.

Devising good multiple choice questions is more difficult for some topics than others, and some questions are themselves more difficult to answer than others. With this in mind, and to help those who wish to use this book as a means of self-assessment, the Appendix provides mean scores and other data on many of the questions, which have been tested on samples of medical students. Some of the questions have been modified after having been tested in this way. In a few instances, we have chosen, because of their importance, to retain questions which remain more ambiguous than they should be in an actual multiple choice examination.

Our intention in writing this book has been to meet the needs of medical undergraduates learning psychiatry and studying for their final qualifying examinations. However, the book will also be useful to junior psychiatric trainees, non-psychiatric doctors studying for postgraduate examinations and others learning psychiatry.

We are very pleased to acknowledge the considerable help and encouragement we received during the preparation of this book from Verity Waite and her colleagues at John Wiley and Sons. Dr Molly McGregor provided valuable help in reading the proofs. We are also indebted to our students, who continue to help us learn how to improve our teaching.

Basic Concepts

MCQ 1

Which of the following statements are true of mental disorders in general?

A. in psychiatry, as in general medicine, disorders are generally classified into different diagnostic groups on the basis of their pathogenesis
B. biochemical and psychological theories of mental disorder are mutually incompatible
C. the principle that one should seek a single cause to account for a patient's illness is a sound basis for psychiatric practice
D. in terms of a person's behaviour or beliefs, all departures from the norms accepted by society are evidence of psychiatric disorder provided that such deviations from the norm are sufficiently extreme
E. anyone who has emotional or psychological problems can be given a psychiatric diagnosis if these problems are sufficiently severe or distressing to bring the person to seek psychiatric help

The 'disease' model in medicine suggests that, associated with every legitimate medical diagnosis, there should be not only signs and symptoms but also a specific underlying pathogenesis. According to this model, every disease is due to some particular abnormality or structure or function of the body. Giving a patient's illness a diagnosis thus implies a particular pathological cause. Superficially at least, this model appears to fit some diagnoses quite well. For example, the diagnosis of a cerebrovascular accident may be made on the history and examination findings, but also implies a particular intracerebral event as its cause. Tuberculosis may be suspected clinically but the diagnosis can be confirmed by the isolation of acid-fast bacilli.

Even in medicine, this 'disease' model often turns out to be simplistic. Not uncommonly, medical diagnosis has little if any relationship with pathogenesis of the illness in question but is based instead on operational criteria, a list of symptoms, signs and investigations, specified combinations of which have to be present to allow the diagnosis to be made. This would have applied, for example, some years ago to diabetes, diagnosed on the basis of clinical presentation together with an arbitrary measure of hyperglycaemia. (More recently, increasing knowledge about diabetes has led to closer links between diagnosis and pathogenesis (insulin-dependent, non-insulin-dependent etc.).) It is naive to think that it is only a matter of time and research before specific pathological causes can be linked with all diagnoses. Even if a specific pathology can be found for any disease, this does not necessarily answer the question how or why the disease manifested itself at a particular time. For example, not all people infected by the tubercle bacillus go on to develop clinical tuberculosis—the pathological agent is *necessary* to cause the illness, but may not be *sufficient*. Such observations have led critics of the 'disease' model to suggest its replacement by a 'biopsychosocial' model of illness, acknowledging the importance of psychological and social factors as well as biological ones in causing illness.

The 'disease' model fits even less successfully in psychiatry, except in a few psychiatric disorders which have a clear organic basis, such as general paresis of the insane (due to syphilis) or Korsakov's psychosis ★. The pathogenesis of most psychiatric disorders is unknown. The development of increasingly sophisticated non-invasive brain imaging techniques, such as positron emission tomography and nuclear magnetic resonance imaging, has revealed that there are specific abnormalities of brain structure or function that correlate with certain psychiatric disorders, notably schizophrenia. Molecular genetics has opened up the possibility of locating particular genes which may be instrumental in the pathogenesis of conditions like schizophrenia and manic depressive psychosis. However, such techniques are likely to confirm that most if not all psychiatric conditions, far from having a single cause, have a complex pathogenesis which involves a multitude of aetiological factors.

Pathological processes can be described in psychological, social, neurological or biochemical terms. Such descriptions are not necessarily mutually exclusive, although some may be more important or relevant than others in understanding individual cases of psychiatric disturbance. Conversely, the same psychiatric syndrome might be usefully described in psychological and biological terms. Thus regular medication with methyldopa and the trauma of early losses in childhood may each predispose to or precipitate a similar depressive illness and, in some cases, both may contribute.

In North America, psychiatric diagnoses are based on operational criteria (see above) specified in the Diagnostic and Statistical Manual, now in the revised form of its third edition (DSM-IIIR). Important criteria include not only the abnormalities of the mental state (the **phenomenology** of the disorder) but also details of the patient's history such as the duration of the illness (a DSM-IIIR diagnosis of schizophrenia, for example, requires that the individual suffer specified symptoms for at least six months). In Europe and elsewhere, the International Classification of Diseases, currently in its 9th edition (ICD9) is used. Unlike DSM-IIIR, the ICD9 is based mainly on phenomenology (thus an ICD9 diagnosis of schizophrenia is not influenced by the duration of the symptoms). Diagnosis and classification are considered further in MCQ 2.

The stigma of mental disorder is an indication that people with psychiatric disorders are commonly seen to deviate from social norms in terms of behaviour, beliefs, etc. However, the converse is certainly not true—departure from a socially accepted norm alone is not necessarily evidence of psychiatric disorder, even when such deviation is extreme. For example, not all multiple murderers can be assigned psychiatric diagnoses. Similarly, it is inappropriate to see all forms of emotional distress as manifestations of psychiatric illness, even when extreme and even when the sufferer presents to a doctor for help. Bereavement is one example of this. FFFFF

The following statements apply to psychiatric diagnosis and classification:

A. assessment of orientation and memory is important in distinguishing organic psychoses from function psychoses
B. the distinction between psychoses and neuroses rests mainly on whether or not the patient has insight into his illness
C. delusions and hallucinations may very occasionally be found in neurotic conditions
D. even a very experienced psychiatrist may have more difficulty in diagnosing some psychiatric disorders than others
E. a patient with a functional psychosis will inevitably also show evidence of a disordered personality

A psychiatric diagnosis represents a description of certain signs and symptoms, based on psychiatric assessment. Often, it also implies that the individual's mental state is likely to follow a particular course and might respond to particular interventions or treatments. There are rules available for classifying psychiatric disorder, notably ICD9 ★ and DSM-IIIR ★.

Although the terms 'diagnosis' and 'classification' are sometimes used interchangeably, they have different meanings. A classification groups patients together on the basis of their similarities. Thus, for example, all those patients classified as schizophrenic have certain features (signs, symptoms, etc.) in common which distinguish them from other patients classified as suffering from manic depressive psychosis. However, schizophrenics are not all alike; differences between individuals with schizophrenia are also very important. For example, an aetiological factor which is important in determining one patient's relapse may be of trivial significance in another case. In the strict sense, diagnosis (or more particularly, the diagnostic formulation) takes such differences into account in attempting to describe in a short-hand form not only the individual's disorder but why it affected him at this particular time in the way that it did.

The distinction between psychosis and neurosis forms an appropriate starting point in psychiatric classification. Traditionally, the distinction between these has been based on the preservation of insight into the illness in neurosis and its absence in psychosis. If a patient can recognise that he is ill and can distinguish clearly between his mental state abnormalities and reality, then he is said to have insight. However, preservation of insight is not as helpful here as it initially appears to be. During the acute phase of a psychotic disorder, it is true that insight is usually lost. However, some patients with schizophrenia (a psychosis) may recognise their auditory hallucinations as 'their voices', different from normal human speech, that is, they may have some degree of insight. In practice, classifying a disorder as a psychosis usually depends on the presence of delusions, hallucinations and/or disorders of the form of thought (MCQ 4–5). These particular mental state abnormalities are hardly ever found except in the psychoses.

Psychoses can be further subdivided into **organic** and **functional**. The main functional psychoses are schizophrenia and manic depressive psychosis. Examples of organic psychoses include dementia ★, Korsakov's psychosis ★ and the acute organic brain syndromes ★. The organic psychoses all involve cognitive abnormalities, like disorientation and impairments of memory and all share a similar aetiology—they are caused by physical illness or **conspicuous** structural and/or functional abnormalities in the brain. These are prerequisites for classifying a disorder as an organic psychosis but are absent in the functional psychoses. It was previously considered that the functional psychoses involved **no** brain changes. However, recent research has started to define specific brain changes which correlate with schizophrenia in particular. However, these changes are subtle compared with those found in the organic psychoses and their precise relevance to the aetiology of the functional psychoses remains unclear (MCQ 37).

In general, psychotic symptoms are not found except as features of psychiatric disorder (but see MCQ 6). Neurotic symptoms, like anxiety, are common in the general population but warrant a psychiatric diagnosis when they are present to an exaggerated extent. Thus psychosis involves qualitative abnormalities, neurosis only quantitative ones. In both cases, however, the abnormalities concerned relate to particular features of the mental state. In personality disorder, the final category in psychiatric classification, such specific mental state abnormalities are commonly absent; personality disorders involve deviation from the norm of the personality as a whole (see MCQ 70). Not surprisingly, psychoses can be classified more reliably than personality disorders—there is better agreement between different psychiatrists in diagnosing someone as demented than as having a personality disorder.

The categories of psychiatric classification described above can be formed into a hierarchy, with organic psychoses at its apex, then schizophrenia, then affective disorder (manic-depressive psychosis, etc.) then the neuroses, and finally personality disorders at the base. Going up this hierarchy, the mental state abnormalities at each level become increasingly specific, first involving deviations from the norm of the personality, then quantitative changes in specific mental state abnormalities, then qualitative changes. If a patient's disorder can be placed at a given level on the hierarchy, the patient will show mental state abnormalities characteristic of that level and of those below it but no abnormalities specific to the levels higher in the hierarchy. For example, schizophrenia is above depression in the hierarchy. Thus a schizophrenic might show evidence of depression (as well as possibly having neurotic symptoms and a disordered personality) but will lack the cognitive abnormalities characterising the organic psychoses, at the top of the hierarchy.

Substance abuse (alcoholism and drug abuse) is rather difficult to locate in this classification (and in the hierarchy) but is usually placed between the neuroses and the personality disorders. TFFTF

MCQ 3

Regarding the mental state examination:

A. compulsions represent a form of stereotypy
B. the patient's *reported* mood can be relied on to agree with features of mood elucidated in the mental state examination
C. ideas of reference represent a type of persecutory delusion
D. an obsession is a recurrent intrusive thought (or idea or image) which the patient recognises as coming from outside himself
E. an overvalued idea is one which for lengthy periods of time takes precedence in the patient's mind over other ideas

In every psychiatric assessment, it is important to go through the mental state examination completely and systematically. Important attributes of the mental state include appearance and behaviour, mood, form and content of speech and thought (including abnormal beliefs), abnormalities of perception and cognition.

Behaviour may be retarded, overactive, agitated, cooperative, etc. There may be evidence of abnormalities of motor function. These include tics (irregular movements of the same group of muscles), mannerisms (repeated movements which appear to have some purpose or function) and stereotypies (repeated movements which have no apparent function or purpose).

In assessing mood, it is important to remember that terms like 'depression' and 'agitation' may mean different things to different individuals. Thus a patient's statement that he feels depressed should not be taken at face value; this should be explored further. In asking about mood, questions must also be included about the 'biological' symptoms ★ of depression.

Speech needs to be assessed in terms of both content (any predominant themes, etc.) and form. Speech may be abnormal in form because of dysarthria (abnormalities in articulation, the mechanical aspects of speech), dysphasia (disruption in verbal expression due to organic brain disease) or formal thought disorder ★.

Abnormal beliefs include delusions ★, overvalued ideas and ideas of reference. An **overvalued idea** is one with which the person is preoccupied—it takes precedence over other thoughts for long periods of time. However, it does not have the properties of a delusion (MCQ 5)—the idea can be understood in terms of the patient's personal or cultural background. Selfconscious people have ideas of reference, which represent a feeling that they are conspicuous and noticed by other people. Those affected realise that these ideas arise in their own minds and are unwarranted. These features distinguish ideas of reference from delusions.

An **obsession** is any 'content of consciousness' like a thought, idea or image, which has a number of specific properties. An obsessional thought, for example, is persistent and recurs. The individual recognises the thought as senseless and often tries to resist it when it comes into his mind. Obsessions differ from delusions in that the person recognises the obsession as his own (coming from within himself) and as abnormal. In other words, insight ★ is preserved, as it is for ideas of reference.

Compulsions are ritualised motor acts which in most cases accompany obsessions, but may also occur alone. They are similar in their features to obsessions in being senseless, recognised as such, etc. As with obsessions, the person often attempts to resist them but then gives in to them. Although compulsions may be stereotyped, they are not strictly speaking stereotypies, because they have features which stereotypies do not share.

Delusions and abnormalities of perception are considered in questions MCQ 5 and MCQ 6.

In assessing the mental state, it is not enough merely to elicit the presence of any of the abnormalities above. The severity of each abnormality, and its impact on the person, are also important. For example, one individual may take an extra five minutes leaving home each day to check several times that the doors and windows are secure; another person might scarcely be able to leave the house because going out involves first getting through five or six hours of washing rituals. Both cases involve obsessions, but the impact of the obsessions is markedly different in the two cases. FFFFT

MCQ 4

Which of the following are examples of formal thought disorder?

A. word salad
B. obsessions
C. neologisms
D. thought alienation
E. Knight's move thinking

'Thought disorder' refers to a number of disparate abnormalities of thought—abnormalities of **stream**, of **content**, of **form** or of **possession** of thought.

The stream of thought may be accelerated—**pressure of thought** (usually manifested as **pressure of speech**). Here, thoughts come very rapidly and may change frequently, moving quickly from one thought to the next. Pressure of thought is often accompanied by flight of ideas (see below); both are particularly associated with mania ★. In depression, poverty of thought may occur—thoughts seem to come to mind slowly. Mutism in depression is an extreme form of this.

Examples of abnormalities of thought content include delusions ★ and obsessions ★.

Formal thought disorder (disorder of the form of thought) refers to the condition in which expected connections between thoughts are obscure or even absent; what the person says may not make sense. The person may jump from one idea to another, even within the same sentence, for example, 'My mother likes strawberries so I want to go home today and I saw a film about motorcycles.' This is known as knight's move thinking, and is a form of loosening of associations. When extreme, speech is completely jumbled up (word salad). Sometimes, the patient will make up new words, either from scratch or possibly by linking together two current words—such new words are called **neologisms**. Loosening of associations can be a feature of schizophrenia. Another type of formal thought disorder, found in mania but also in schizophrenia, is **flight of ideas**. The person jumps from one idea to the next very rapidly. The ideas may be connected not by concepts but by particular words which rhyme forming part of successive pieces of speech—this is known as clang association.

Disorders of possession of thought involve **thought alienation**, in which the patient experiences others controlling or participating in his thoughts. Examples include **thought withdrawal** (in which the patient believes that thoughts are withdrawn from his mind), **thought broadcast** (in which the patient believes that his thoughts are being broadcast to others, over the radio or television, for example), and **thought insertion** (thoughts being put into the person's mind). These are all types of passivity experience, and may be found in schizophrenics. They constitute Schneiderian first-rank symptoms ★.

The term 'thought disorder' thus embraces several disparate phenomena. Most of these phenomena have more specific names (delusions, pressure of thought, etc.) and for these, there is nothing to be gained by using 'thought disorder'. To say that someone has 'thought disorders' could mean that he is severely obsessional, very deluded or even mute. It is probably best to confine use of the term to formal thought disorder. TFTFT

Which of the following statements are true of delusions?

A. delusions are unshakeable beliefs held for inappropriate or inadequate reasons
B. delusions are always false
C. patients with genuine delusions usually act in accordance with their delusions
D. a primary delusion arises in a manner that is not understandably related to prior abnormal perceptions, thought or mood
E. delusions are usually incongruent with mood

Delusions are abnormal beliefs, not in keeping with the patient's social and cultural background, held with unshakeable conviction but for inadequate or inappropriate reasons. What determines whether an idea is a delusion is not the form of the idea nor its content, but the nature of the patient's belief in the idea. Often, there is evidence against the idea, but this is not always the case— delusions are not necessarily false. For example, a man may be convinced that his wife is having an affair with a neighbour. His entire evidence for this is that on one occasion when he (the patient) was coming home, he noticed the light in their bedroom being turned on at the same time as the neighbour's bedroom light. Further questioning fails to elucidate the meaning of this evidence, beyond the patient's claim that his wife and his neighbour were obviously signalling to one another. This belief is a delusion, whether or not his wife *is* having an affair, because it is held for an inadequate and probably inappropriate reason. This particular delusion, sometimes a feature of **morbid jealousy**, is important because when it occurs, there is a serious risk that the person might act on it, putting his wife at risk. In general, however, it is not possible to predict reliably whether or not a patient is likely to act on his delusions. The belief has to be considered in the light of past and current behaviour. In some cases, especially among chronic schizophrenic patients, a patient's actions can be quite incongruent with his delusional beliefs. For example, a patient may believe he is a member of the royal family and yet make no effort to alter his menial lifestyle.

In some instances, it is relatively easy to demonstrate the inappropriateness of a person's convictions regarding his delusions. However, this is not always so. For example, extreme religious beliefs are not necessarily delusional if they are held by others of the same culture as the patient.

Sometimes, delusions are secondary to other mental state abnormalities. For example, a man who hears persecutory voices may develop the delusional belief that certain people are attempting to harm him. Similarly, a depressed patient might believe that his sins will be the cause of a nuclear holocaust. In depression and mania, the content of delusions is usually congruent with mood—in schizophrenia, delusions are often not congruent with mood. Some delusions arise out of nothing, often as a sudden conviction, in a manner quite inconsistent with prior abnormal perceptions, thought or mood. For example, a man might see a dog in the street and become convinced that he has a special mission to save the world. These are called primary delusions, which are a Schneiderian first-rank symptom ★.

Delusions, together with hallucinations, are cardinal features of all the psychoses (MCQ 2). TFFTF

Hallucinations:

A. are perceptions experienced in the absence of a related stimulus to a sensory organ
B. which occur in organic psychoses are often visual
C. differ from illusions in that the latter involve a genuine sensory stimulus
D. differ from pseudohallucinations in that the latter are forms of abnormal belief rather than abnormal perception
E. only occur in people who are mentally ill

Hallucinations and illusions are both disorders of perception. Hallucinations are percepts not based on stimulation of a sensory organ. In illusions, there is a sensory stimulus leading to the perception, but the perception is distorted, sometimes dramatically so. Thus a patient might gaze at a wall, look at an electric cable running up it and perceive a snake. Illusions occur particularly in organic psychoses.

It is possible to experience hallucinations in any sensory modality, but auditory and visual hallucinations are the most common. In acute organic brain syndromes, visual hallucinations are the most common. In schizophrenia and depression, auditory hallucinations are the most typical, although visual, olfactory and tactile hallucinations can occur. The content of hallucinations is often helpful diagnostically, especially when considered in the light of the patient's mood. In manic-depressive psychosis (bipolar affective disorder), hallucinations are often mood-congruent.

Despite their relevance in psychiatric diagnosis, hallucinations can occur in people who are not mentally ill. They are particularly likely to occur at the point of falling asleep (hypnagogic hallucinations) or awakening (hypnopompic hallucinations). They also occur during bereavement.

There are two definitions of pseudohallucinations. The first is that these are hallucinations into which the patient has insight. The problem with this definition is that psychotic patients not uncommonly acquire insight into their mental state abnormalities as treatment proceeds. Thus one would end up calling a particular abnormal perception an hallucination one day and a pseudohallucination the next. The other definition of pseudohallucinations is that they arise within the head. This contrasts with hallucinations, which appear to the patient just like real percepts, arising in outside space and being 'received' through the appropriate sense organ. Thus an auditory hallucination will be heard exactly like any other voice, outside the patient's body, and will be 'heard' through the ears. An auditory pseudohallucination will be heard coming from within the head. This second definition of pseudohallucination is preferable to the first. Whatever definition is adopted, pseudohallucinations are a type of abnormal perception rather than an abnormal belief. In practice, it may in any case be difficult to distinguish pseudohallucinations from hallucinations. TTTFF

Which of the following statements about the cognitive examination are true?

A. disorientation in person (not knowing who one is) is a sensitive indicator of clouding of consciousness
B. disorientation in time is more frequently encountered than disorientation in place
C. the serial sevens test is purely a measure of concentration
D. reciting the months of the year backwards is a test of attention
E. in assessing attention, it is usually adequate to rely on the patient's behaviour during the interview

It is customary to begin the cognitive examination by assessing orientation, because disorientation is a measure of clouding of consciousness, associated with the organic brain syndromes. Other cognitive tests require unimpaired consciousness to allow their accurate interpretation. The patient's orientation is assessed in terms of time, place and person. Of these, the last is the least sensitive—orientation in time is usually the first to be affected by impaired consciousness. Remember that a patient who has been in hospital for some time may not have access to the usual cues about time (like newspapers or calendars) and thus might have difficulty recalling the exact day or date without necessarily being disorientated. However, more likely indicators of disorientation include not knowing what season it is (or what month), being unable to remember whether the last meal was breakfast or dinner, and not knowing the approximate time of day (providing that appropriate cues are present like natural light, visiting times and mealtimes).

The distinction between attention and concentration is subtle and not particularly important clinically. It is possible to gain some idea of the patient's attention by merely observing what happens in the interview—Is the patient distractible? Does his mind appear to stray from the interview? And so on. However, it is useful to try to quantify this, particularly because changes in attention and concentration may be important clinically (in acute organic brain syndromes, for example—MCQ 14). The difficulty of the test can be adjusted to suit the patient's mental state and also to take into account other factors like intelligence. A common test is to ask the patient to subtract 7 from 100 then subtract 7 from the answer and so on, recording the time in seconds it takes to reach 2 and the number of mistakes made. This is the serial sevens test. A grocer (or someone accustomed to mental arithmetic) may be more skilled at this task than others. Someone of low intelligence might find this test too difficult—serial threes can be used instead. Easier tests involve asking the patient to recite the months of the year backwards from December, or the days of the week from Saturday. If the patient's attention is too poor even to achieve this, the patient can be asked to count down from 100, or even up from one. FTFTF

Which of the following are appropriate tests of recent memory?

A. immediate recall of a name and address
B. recall of the interviewer's name at the end of the interview
C. immediate recall of at least five digits forwards in the digit span test
D. recall of three unconnected words after five minutes
E. knowing the names of the current prime minister and monarch

Clinically, it is useful to classify memory into three components—immediate memory, recent memory and remote memory. Other functions important in memory are registration and recall.

The capacity to form new memories is dependent on attention and concentration—if these are impaired (as in an acute organic brain syndrome, for example), memory is difficult to test. Thus it is helpful in the cognitive examination to test attention and concentration (MCQ 7) before testing memory.

Immediate memory covers little more than registration of new memories and spans seconds rather than minutes. It may be measured using the digit span test. The patient is given a series of numbers (with progressively more digits) and instructed to repeat them back to the interviewer. The patient is given longer numbers until he reaches a number of digits at which he makes more than one mistake—the digit span is the highest number of digits the patient can repeat back. It is very important not to say the numbers too quickly—try to leave a gap of about a second between digits, because this makes the results more consistent. If the interviewer presents the digits too quickly, they are easier to remember (think of remembering a telephone number by grouping the digits—this is easier to do if the digits are presented in quick succession). An additional test, more difficult than this, is the reverse digit span, in which the interviewer again gives the patient progressively longer numbers but this time asks the patient to repeat them backwards. Immediate recall of a name and address would also be a test of immediate memory.

Recent memory involves recall of memories within minutes rather than days. Commonly, the patient is taught a name and address, and told that he will be asked for it again in five minutes. In the intervening time, other cognitive tests can be done. After five minutes, the patient's recollection is recorded exactly in the notes. It is important to make sure the patient has learnt the name and address to begin with, otherwise recollection after five minutes is bound to be inaccurate. If the patient has difficulty learning the address, the interviewer can also record how many trials were necessary before the address was learnt. Alternatively, the patient can be asked to remember three unconnected words such as 'daisy spoon purple' and then asked what the words are after five minutes.

Remote memory is usually tested using questions about general knowledge which most people should be able to answer (for example, someone who lived through the Second World War is likely to remember the year it started and the year it ended, and also the name of one prime minister during the war). The consistency of a patient's personal history can also give some clues regarding remote memory.

13

These memory tests should form part of every mental state assessment. Beyond them, there are more sophisticated tests used under special circumstances. For example, the tests described above relate mainly to verbal memory—there are equivalent tests to assess non-verbal memory.

All this relates to the *clinical* assessment of memory, relevant to the psychiatric mental state. It is worth noting that neuropsychologists have somewhat different, and more sophisticated, models of memory, and may also use the terms 'recent' and 'remote' differently. FTFTF

Regarding the epidemiology of psychiatric disorders:

A. the prevalence of most psychiatric disorders is higher in women than in men
B. most psychiatric disorders are equally prevalent across the social classes
C. in general, immigrants show psychiatric disorders less commonly than does the indigenous population
D. psychiatric disorders among patients attending psychiatric outpatients or admitted to psychiatric units form a representative sample of psychiatric disturbance in the population as a whole
E. the cultural or ethnic background of the psychiatrist may influence significantly the psychiatric diagnoses he makes

With relatively few exceptions, the prevalence of particular psychiatric disorders in adults is greater in women than in men (this is different in children—see MCQ 98). Multi-infarct dementia ★ is more common among men than women (or at least has been until recently). Alcoholism ★ and psychopathic personality ★ are more common in males. Suicide is also more common among men, although deliberate self-harm ★ is more prevalent among women. Below the age of 35, schizophrenia is more prevalent among males but beyond this age, the reverse is true. Disorders which are not significantly more common in either sex include obsessional compulsive neurosis ★, social phobia ★ and manic depressive psychosis (bipolar affective disorder ★). Note that unipolar affective disorder is more prevalent among women than men.

Some psychiatric disorders are equally prevalent in all socioeconomic groups—Alzheimer-type senile dementia ★ is one example. However, many disorders do show an unequal social class distribution. Where this occurs, as a general rule, prevalence is higher in the lower socioeconomic groups. However, there are some exceptions—it is commonly held that anorexia nervosa is more prevalent among the higher social classes. Bipolar affective disorder has also been reported to have a higher prevalence in the higher social classes, but this has not been a consistent finding in research studies. Two main models have been proposed to account for the higher prevalence of most psychiatric disorders in the lower socioeconomic classes. One hypothesis suggests that many of the factors which are important in predisposing to or precipitating psychiatric illness, like stressful life events, unemployment and poor social support, are more common in the lower socioeconomic groups. The 'drift' hypothesis (which has been applied particularly to schizophrenia) proposes that, regardless of their original socioeconomic status, people who develop psychiatric disorders tend to drift down the social ladder and thus accumulate in the lower socioeconomic groups. In practice, both of these models apply, but possibly to differing degrees in individual cases.

Provided that rigorous diagnostic criteria are used, the prevalence of major psychiatric disorders, notably schizophrenia and affective disorder, can be shown to be remarkably similar across different cultures. However, the ethnic and cultural background (both of the patient and the psychiatrist) can have a profound effect on the manifestation and detection of psychiatric disorders. Some cultures discriminate more accurately than others between different types of emotion (anger, irritability, sadness, etc.). In some cultures, people tend to 'translate' emotions into bodily feelings (an example might be to suffer a 'heavy heart')—this is termed **somatisation**. In this respect, it is interesting that there are more words available to describe unpleasant emotions in most Indo-European languages than in some others. Unless the psychiatrist is familiar with his patient's cultural background, he can misinterpret what the patient is trying to convey about his bodily feelings. Thus the psychiatrist's background may influence his appraisal of his patients.

In England, people of West Indian origin are less likely than indigenous people to commit suicide, but have a much higher rate of inpatient admissions for schizophrenia and a lower admission rate for alcoholism. People born in Germany, living in England, have approximately the same rates of hospital admission for alcoholism and schizophrenia as those born in England, but a much higher suicide rate. These observations illustrate the complex effects of migration on psychiatric morbidity, effects which depend on many factors including ethnic and cultural background, the reason for migration, time away from country of origin, etc. An added complication is that the presentation of psychiatric disorders in immigrants may show 'atypical' features, possibly leading to inaccuracies in diagnosis unless adequate care is taken. For example, the higher admission rate for schizophrenia among West Indians can partly be accounted for by the occurrence among New Commonwealth immigrants in particular of an atypical functional psychosis, with acute onset, dramatic presentation (often requiring compulsory admission) and often religious overtones. It is likely in the past that such psychoses were diagnosed as schizophrenia, although this may not be justified, as these atypical psychoses are characteristically short-lived and have a much better prognosis compared with schizophrenia as a whole.

Hospital admission rates (or even psychiatric outpatient clinic statistics) give a biased picture of psychiatric morbidity, because only the more severely disordered patients come to psychiatric attention (see MCQ 109). TFFFT

Regarding the aetiology of psychiatric disorders:

A. the fact that a particular psychiatric disorder runs within families is strong evidence that the disorder has a genetic basis
B. a higher concordance of a given psychiatric disorder in monozygous twins than in dizygous twins may be explained by an increased incidence of the disorder in monozygous twins compared with others
C. genetic factors are more important in manic depressive psychosis than in obsessive-compulsive neurosis
D. genetic evidence provides the only significant data supporting the important contribution of biological factors to the aetiology of the functional psychoses
E. many psychiatric disorders are associated with particular types of body build (physique)

All psychiatric disorders show complex aetiology, involving biological, psychological and social components.

That a particular condition runs in families does not alone suggest that a genetic component is important aetiologically. For example, many parents who abuse their children were themselves abused in childhood. Here, family environment may be important, whatever the contribution of genetic factors. More convincing evidence of a genetic contribution to a particular disorder may be gained from studies of twins and adoptees.

In twin studies, the concordance for a particular disorder within twin pairs can be measured—this estimates the likelihood, if one twin has the disorder in question, of the other twin also being affected. Concordance among monozygotic twins is compared with that among dizygotic twins. Remembering that the genetic makeup of monozygotic twins is identical while dizygotic twins share only half their genes, a higher concordance among monozygotic twins than their dizygotic counterparts suggests a genetic contribution to aetiology. If the concordances are similar (despite the difference in shared genes), this offers evidence against an important genetic contribution. Thus the concordance for schizophrenia has been estimated as 50% for monozygotic twins and 12% for dizygotic twins. One could argue that being one of an identical twin pair itself predisposes to schizophrenia. However, this would lead to the prediction of a higher *prevalence* as well as concordance of schizophrenia among monozygotic twins—this is not the case. Besides, concordance remains similar, even if the twins are reared apart.

From adoption studies, it is clear that the incidence of schizophrenia is higher among the children of schizophrenic parents, even when these children were adopted away from their natural parents soon after birth. By contrast, children born to non-schizophrenic parents and adopted away at an equally early age, whose adoptive parents have or go on to develop schizophrenia, show no greater incidence of schizophrenia than that found in the general population.

A genetic component has been established for a number of psychiatric disorders, including schizophrenia, affective disorder, Alzheimer-type senile dementia, alcohol dependence and some of the neuroses. In general, the genetic contribution to aetiology (termed 'genetic loading') is greater for the functional psychoses (schizophrenia and affective disorder) than for the neuroses, and probably less important for personality disorders.

Apart from such genetic data, other evidence supports the contribution of biological factors to the aetiology of psychiatric disorders, notably the functional psychoses. For example, use of amphetamines can produce a mental state resembling that in schizophrenia (a **schizophreniform** psychosis ★) and a wide variety of commonly prescribed drugs has been implicated in contributing to depression, including some beta-blockers, sulphonamides, l-dopa and steroids. The fact that many effective anti-psychotic drugs block the postsynaptic reuptake of dopamine has led to much research into the possible role of dopamine in schizophrenia. The same applies to other monoamines (notably noradrenaline and 5-hydroxytryptamine) in depression—most effective antidepressants have effects on either or both of these neurotransmitters. However, despite much effort, no satisfactory biological or physiological markers have been established for any of the common psychiatric disorders, further evidence for the complexity of their aetiology.

In the past, it was commonly held that many psychiatric disorders, like schizophrenia and depression, were associated with certain types of physique. There is no evidence to support this idea in general, although physique may be very important in some specific psychiatric syndromes, such as anorexia nervosa ★. FFTFF

Regarding the aetiology of psychiatric disorders:

A. it has been well established that particular personality types are associated with the subsequent development of a number of psychiatric disorders
B. as a factor possibly contributing to psychiatric illness, loss of a pet dog should always be regarded as less important than loss of a spouse
C. a person who is married is more likely than someone who is single to develop any psychiatric disorder
D. sufficiently careful examination of any psychiatric disorder will reveal particular aetiological factors which are shared by most if not all people with that diagnosis.
E. for adult psychiatric disorders in general, childhood experiences play a major aetiological role

Life events can play a major role in predisposing to or precipitating psychiatric disorders and also some types of physical illness (MCQ 107). For example, in schizophrenia, patients who relapse show a higher frequency of stressful life events shortly before readmission to hospital than at other times. In the case of schizophrenia, such life events need not have negative impact on the individual to have the effect—positive events can also precipitate acute symptoms. By contrast, life events which precede depression are negative (like significant losses) or may represent chronic difficulties. It is not the life event itself but its significance to the individual that is important. Thus the loss of a pet dog may mean just as much to a single, isolated animal lover as the loss of a close personal friend or spouse might to others.

Social supports can serve an important protective function against the development of psychiatric disorder. However, their influence is complex. The extent of a person's social network is important, but so also is the quality of the relationships involved. The contribution of each of these in limiting psychiatric morbidity is likely to vary from one person to the next. Thus a happy marriage may be a strong source of support, while an unsatisfactory relationship with a spouse or partner may be a source of considerable stress. Also, social supports may have different effects for men and women.

Psychoanalytic theory suggests that the mental health of adults should be considerably affected by childhood experiences. That this is the case can sometimes be demonstrated in individual cases, during psychoanalysis for example. However, research has so far failed in its attempts to demonstrate a major aetiological role in the common adult psychiatric disorders of specific events in childhood. There is evidence that the loss of one's mother in early childhood predisposes some women to depression in adulthood, but this has not been a universal finding. The same applies to personality types. While some people who develop obsessional compulsive neurosis, for example, may have been obsessional all their lives, there is no clear evidence that having an obsessional personality serves as a significant risk factor in the development of obsessional compulsive neurosis. Although there is an association between neurotic traits in childhood (like enuresis ★) and adult neurotic disorders, this is not an important aetiological factor. The majority of adults with neurosis showed no evidence of neurotic traits as children, and most children with neurotic traits do not go on to develop neurotic disorders in adulthood.

In general, it is not possible to isolate particular aetiological factors shared by all patients with a particular psychiatric disorder. Thus, for example, the fact that a group of patients with schizophrenia share the same mental state abnormalities does not imply that the aetiology of the disorder is the same in each case, or even similar. Even when a psychiatric disorder apparently involves one major aetiological factor (as, for example, in post-natal psychosis ★) the clinical picture is not as clear-cut as it seems. That most women do not develop post-natal psychosis after childbirth indicates that other aetiological factors must also play an important part. FFFFF

Organic Disorders

MCQ 12

The following statements apply to organic psychiatric disorders:

A. disturbance of cognitive function is characteristic
B. focal neurological signs are always present
C. memory is always impaired
D. symptoms of a schizophrenic illness make the diagnosis of an organic disorder very unlikely
E. some psychiatric disorders have a definite organic aetiology without giving rise to cognitive impairment

The main feature characteristic of organic disorders is impairment of cognition. **Cognition** refers to mental processes concerned with thinking, perception, memory, language and fine movement. It reflects central as opposed to peripheral neuronal activity and abnormalities of cognitive function reflect central nervous system pathology. It is important to note, however, that some psychiatric disorders may have a definite organic aetiology without necessarily giving rise to cognitive impairment (amphetamine abuse, for example, can give rise to a psychosis resembling schizophrenia). Besides impaired cognition, the organic disorders may involve the whole gamut of mental symptoms, including delusions, hallucinations and affective symptoms (see MCQ 2).

Organic psychiatric disorders may be classified according to their pattern of cognitive impairment. This may be focal of diffuse, reflecting the underlying pattern of brain pathology.

Focal brain pathology may give rise to circumscribed cognitive deficits, reflecting the functions of the brain region affected. Such focal cognitive abnormalities include disturbances of speech (dysphasia), memory (amnesia), perception (agnosia), writing (dysgraphia), reading (dyslexia), arithmetical abilities (dyscalculia) and the execution of coordinated movements (dyspraxia).

Where brain pathology is more widespread, cognitive impairment follows a more diffuse pattern, with more widely ranging deficits apparent. Such a pattern is seen in acute brain syndromes ★ and in a group of disorders giving rise to the syndrome of dementia ★.

Organic psychiatric disorders are sometimes accompanied by focal neurological signs, but these are not present in every case. TFFFT

Impairment of recent memory is characteristic of:

A. schizophrenia
B. bilateral hippocampal lesions
C. dementia
D. transient global amnesia
E. depressive pseudodementia

Impairment of recent memory (MCQ 8) is present in a wide variety of organic psychiatric disorders. Organic disorders of memory can be divided into two types depending upon whether the underlying brain pathology is focal or diffuse. Focal lesions in certain specific areas of the brain may lead to amnesic deficits which are relatively discrete and not associated with parallel deterioration of other cognitive functions. Diffuse pathology on the other hand produces amnesic deficits which are accompanied by a more general cognitive deterioration. This latter picture is characteristic of dementia.

Two regions of the brain are particularly important in relation to memory. These are the hypothalamic-diencephalic region and the hippocampal region of the temporal lobe. Lesions in either of these relatively discrete areas will selectively impair recent memory. Severe memory loss is only seen however when the lesions are bilateral. Such lesions are also associated with a period of retrograde amnesia of variable duration but remote memory remains un-affected. Thus, for example, someone with focal seizures may recall what led up to a seizure and may have some recollection of the seizure itself, unless the epileptic discharge involved both temporal lobes.

Causes of lesions in the hypothalamic-diencephalic region include thiamine deficiency, subarachnoid haemorrhage, tumour and meningovascular syphilis. Such lesions can give rise to the clinical picture of **Korsakoff's psychosis** ★. This is characterised by impairment of memory (especially recent memory) and a disordered sense of time. The patient characteristically shows 'islets' of pre-served memory but may not be able to put these memories into the right time sequence. Thus he may accurately recall a remote event but describe it as though it happened recently. Gaps in memory may be filled by making the details up—confabulation. Bilateral hippocampal lesions are rare and are most commonly due to herpes encephalitis.

Transient global amnesia is an uncommon syndrome characterised by abrupt episodes of severe short-term memory loss with full preservation of conscious-ness and other cognitive functions. Attacks may last for several hours, then resolve fully. There may be a retrograde amnesia for weeks or rarely years but remote memory and personal identity are preserved. Patients commonly display anxious bewilderment. The disorder is attributed in most cases to transient ischaemia of the hippocampal and hypothalamic areas.

Impaired memory is not a characteristic feature of functional psychiatric illnesses. However, in the elderly especially, it may be difficult to distinguish depression from dementia. Cognitive assessment of an elderly depressed person may reveal deficits suggestive of dementia, even in the absence of significant brain pathology. However, these deficits are not always consistent on reassessment, and respond, along with the other depressive symptoms, to appropriate treatment for depression. This syndrome is known as **depressive pseudodementia** ★. Another distinction between this and dementia which is sometimes helpful is that pseudodementia rarely involves clearly defined temporoparietal abnormalities such as dysphasia, dyslexia and agnosia.

Impaired recent memory or other cognitive deficits are not characteristic of schizophrenia. Finding cognitive abnormalities in a schizophrenic should raise the suspicion of an organic disorder. However, it has become increasingly recognised that a proportion of chronic schizophrenics do display an impairment of cognitive function which may be associated with enlargement of the lateral cerebral ventricles. FTTTT

Acute brain syndromes:

A. all share the same common and specific pathological process
B. are irreversible
C. characteristically involve impairment of consciousness
D. are not usually associated with impairment of attention
E. are always associated with delusions and/or hallucinations

Acute brain syndrome (also known as **acute confusional state** or **acute organic reaction**) is a term used to describe the symptoms produced by a great number of pathological processes affecting the brain. These processes may be local or systemic and include infection, trauma, anoxia, epilepsy, metabolic disorders and the toxic effects of drugs or alcohol. The onset of symptoms is commonly abrupt and usually reversible when the underlying pathology can be remedied.

The cardinal clinical feature of the syndrome is impairment of consciousness—global impairment of cognitive functioning together with reduced awareness of the environment. In some instances, impairment of consciousness may be extreme, as in coma, severe head injury or in some post-ictal states. More commonly, the change is more subtle, and elicited only by careful cognitive examination. Clinically, it is often helpful to assess orientation, which is impaired in the acute brain syndromes. In addition, evidence may be elicited of impaired attention and concentration as well as memory disturbance.

Other symptoms which may also be present include behavioural abnormalities (like agitation or restlessness) and disturbances of speech, emotion, thought and perception. Certain causes of acute brain syndromes may produce insomnia and agitation while other causes lead to lethargy, hypersomnia and sleep inversion. Speech may be fragmented or incoherent. Emotions may be blunted, but extreme fear and false jocularity may be encountered in response to illusions and hallucinations, which often dominate the clinical picture although they are not invariably present. The abnormal perceptions are characteristically visual and/or somatic, but other modalities may be affected. Delusions may be present but these are usually fleeting and not well elaborated as in the functional psychoses; they are usually secondary to abnormalities of perception (illusions and hallucinations).

Another characteristic of the acute brain syndromes, particularly when clouding of consciousness is mild, is that the symptoms fluctuate. A patient who is disoriented at one time may appear lucid a short time later. The symptoms are particularly likely to manifest when the patient is tired or when there is decreased environmental stimulation. Thus patients with acute brain syndromes commonly become more disturbed at night. FFTFF

MCQ 15

The following are invariably acute brain syndromes:

A. delirium
B. stupor
C. confusion
D. Wernicke's encephalopathy
E. alcoholic withdrawal syndrome (delirium tremens)

In the past, acute brain syndromes were sometimes termed (acute) confusional states. Unfortunately, the term 'confusion' has a very different meaning in lay terms than the acute brain syndrome. Saying that a patient is confused does not necessarily imply that he is, for example, disoriented. Because of its different meanings, it is best to avoid this term in clinical practice.

Stupor, like confusion, has several different meanings and is thus difficult to apply in clinical practice. In the past, the term has been used to describe a form of impaired consciousness, but its use in this context is redundant and should be avoided. It is best to regard stupor as defining the syndrome comprising akinesia (lack of movement) and mutism but with preservation of consciousness. It has a variety of causes, including severe depression (psychomotor retardation might manifest as **depressive stupor**) and schizophrenia (catatonic stupor). Where akinesia and mutism are caused by an organic brain syndrome, they are accompanied by impairment of consciousness.

Delirium has been used synonymously with the acute brain syndrome, but its use is best reserved for those acute brain syndromes in which, in addition to impairment of consciousness, there are conspicuous abnormalities of affect (like lability, fear or irritability) and perception (illusions and/or hallucinations). According to this definition, all cases of delirium are acute brain syndromes, but not all acute brain syndromes cause delirium. The alcohol withdrawal syndrome (delirium tremens) ★ is a form of acute brain syndrome which follows shortly after withdrawal from excessive alcohol consumption. It characteristically starts within hours after the last drink, with tremulousness, insomnia, nausea, sweating and irritability, often accompanied by fear. Many of these symptoms are manifestations of autonomic over-arousal. Illusions and hallucinations, commonly visual, are often very vivid. The condition requires acute and active medical management (see Clinical Case 2).

Wernicke's encephalopathy ★ is an acute brain syndrome resulting from thiamine deficiency. This is characterised by the triad of acute brain syndrome, ataxia and ophthalmoplegia, although these three features may not be present at the same time. Apathy and impaired memory are common, although disturbances of perception less so. The condition generally responds to treatment with parenteral thiamine, although patients may be left with residual ataxia and/or horizontal nystagmus. Some patients are left with Korsakoff's psychosis ★. TFFTT

Regarding acute brain syndromes:

A. they often have multiple causes
B. they have pathogonomic EEG changes which can confirm the diagnosis
C. after dementia is established they occur less frequently
D. sedation is the most important part of management
E. the patient is best nursed in a dimly-lit room

Acute brain syndromes often have multiple causes, especially in the elderly. In someone who is demented, an acute brain syndrome may follow a relatively minor disturbance or disruption, such as removal from a familiar environment or even constipation. An important iatrogenic cause of acute brain syndrome is polytherapy with prescribed drugs, to which the elderly may again be particularly susceptible.

The major aim in the management of an acute brain syndrome is to find and treat its underlying cause, which, by definition, will be organic. Full physical examination is necessary, with particular attention to the neurological system. Because the clinical picture is likely to fluctuate (MCQ 14), repeated and regular monitoring of the cognitive state might be necessary to make or confirm the diagnosis.

This should be followed by appropriate investigations suggested by the clinical presentation and examination findings. Where the diagnosis is unclear, an EEG may be helpful, because if this is well within normal limits, the diagnosis of acute brain syndrome is suspect. Under some circumstances, the EEG might also offer information about possible causes of the syndrome, for example when focal abnormalities are present. More commonly, the EEG shows diffuse and relatively non-specific changes. There is no specific EEG abnormality associated with acute brain syndromes.

In addition to finding and (if possible) treating the cause(s) of the organic syndrome, management might need to incorporate symptomatic treatment if, for example, the patient becomes excessively disturbed. Here, sedation may be appropriate, remembering that this can only 'dampen down' the symptoms rather than deal with their cause. In general, antipsychotic drugs may be used to alleviate distress and disturbed behaviour, both of which may be present when abnormal perceptual experiences are prominent. Caution is necessary, however, because these drugs further depress the level of consciousness. As a rule, benzodiazepines should be avoided because they cause disinhibition and have a tendency to produce paradoxical aggression. However, in the alcohol and barbiturate withdrawal syndromes, there is a risk of withdrawal fits and here benzodiazepines or equivalent drugs are useful in view of their anticonvulsant properties.

Patients are best managed in a bright, evenly-lit room, with changes of environment kept to a minimum. Such measures avoid environmental ambiguity and reduce the occurrence of illusions and the paranoid interpretation of events. Also important are regular observations of conscious state and vital signs, and attention to nutrition, fluid and electrolyte balance and pressure areas. TFFFF

Clinical features of dementia include:

A. impairment of consciousness
B. personality deterioration
C. delusions
D. perseveration
E. incontinence

Dementia refers to a clinical syndrome characterised by the progressive disintegration of intellect and personality together with diffuse impairment of memory and other specific cognitive functions.

The condition usually has an insidious onset (but see MCQ 19), although it may come to light acutely, for example when a supportive spouse falls ill and is admitted to hospital, and the dementing person is no longer able to cope alone. There is commonly evidence in the history of progressive difficulties coping with everyday activities. Early signs may include loss of initiative, a decline in personal standards or episodes of being muddled. Later, embarrassing or dangerous lapses of behaviour may occur, such as wandering and getting lost, neglecting nutrition and personal hygiene, undressing or urinating in public, or screaming and aggressiveness.

Changes in personality include deterioration of manners and a progressive insensitivity to the needs and feelings of others. Loss of normal personal restraints may lead to stealing or disinhibited sexual behaviour. Longstanding personality traits such as anxiety, depression or suspiciousness may be exacerbated.

In their behaviour, some patients will display insomnia and restless anxiety while others are withdrawn and inactive. Affect may be blunted or alternatively depression and anxiety may be present. Emotional lability may be marked with outbursts of anger, hostility or tearfulness, particularly when the person becomes frustrated in his failure in a particular task—this is called the **catastrophic reaction**. Conversation often involves a limited number of themes and ideas which are commonly shallow—**poverty of thought**. There may be **perseveration**, with the patient repeatedly returning to a given topic when the conversation has moved to further topics.

Symptoms of functional psychiatric illness may be present, such as delusions and hallucinations. Such symptoms may occasionally dominate the clinical picture, in which case only careful examination of the cognitive state will reveal the underlying intellectual deterioration.

Cognitive state examination reveals global impairment of intellect. Memory loss is often the most obvious specific cognitive deficit but the pattern of cognitive impairment is diffuse and other specific deficits, such as dysphasia, agnosia and dyspraxia may also be present. Memory loss is most marked for recent events. Impairment of consciousness is not a feature of dementia itself, but occurs in acute brain syndromes to which the demented person is prone. Note that the demented person is likely not to know the correct time of day or where he is, but such disorientation is not due to impaired consciousness but rather to memory deficits.

As the dementia progresses, epilepsy, parkinsonism, incontinence of urine and faeces and focal neurological signs may develop. In the latter stages purposive activity declines, mannerisms and stereotypies develop, and death follows physical deterioration. FTTTT

MCQ 18

Senile dementia of the Alzheimer type (SDAT):

A. is more common in women than men
B. only occurs before the age of 65
C. shows pathology largely confined to the frontal lobe
D. runs in families
E. shows evidence of a viral aetiolgy

Senile dementia of the Alzheimer type (SDAT) is the most common cause of dementia in old age. Historically, senile dementia has been distinguished from Alzheimer's disease, the most common cause of dementia before the age of 65 (but much less common than SDAT). However, the two conditions show very similar brain pathology, hence the term Alzheimer-type senile dementia. However, age of onset may influence the clinical course of the condition—Alzheimer's disease is associated with more marked involvement of the temporal and parietal lobes and a more rapid deterioration. There is some evidence that in SDAT, parietal lobe involvement is associated with a worse prognosis. Women are more commonly affected than men in both conditions.

The precise aetiology of both Alzheimer's disease and SDAT is obscure, but it is recognised that first-degree relatives of sufferers are four times more likely to develop the disease thatn the general population. There are currently two main schools of thought regarding the neurochemical correlates of SDAT. One view is that the disorder is related to abnormalities in cholinergic neurones. Such abnormalities, which include reductions in the enzymes choline acetyl transferase and acetyl cholinesterase, have been related to the severity of the disorder. Such observations have led to attempts at treatment, using acetylcholine precursors. However, such treatments have been largely unsuccessful to date. The other suggestion is that the neurochemical changes are far less specific and embrace many different neurotransmitter systems. Whether these changes are of aetiological significance or secondary phenomena is unclear, whichever model applies. There is no evidence that SDAT is caused by a virus.

Pathologically the disease is characterised by generalised brain atrophy, with particularly marked involvement of the cerebral cortex. All cortical regions are involved but the frontal and temporal lobes are often particularly affected. The cerebral ventricles are enlarged, sulci widened and gyri narrowed.

Histologically there is severe nerve cell loss with secondary gliosis. Senile plaques and neurofibrillary tangles are present, the latter usually being regarded as essential for diagnosis. Senile plaques consist of abnormal neuronal processes intermingled with astrocytes or microglia. Larger plaques may contain amyloid. Neurofibrillary tangles are abnormal intracellular structures consisting of aggregated bundles of filaments within the perikaryon of pyramidal neurones. TFFTF

Multi-infarct dementia:

A. is recognised to have a genetic component to its aetiology
B. is commonly associated with systemic hypertension
C. and Alzheimer-type senile dementia frequently coexist
D. is characterised by a 'step-wise' deterioration
E. is commonly punctuated by episodes of acute brain syndrome

Multi-infarct dementia was previously called atherosclerotic dementia; the former term is preferable because it is more accurate. This type of dementia is caused by cerebral infarction—atherosclerosis contributes to this process but on its own does not give rise to dementia. Given this aetiology, it is not surprising that patients with mult-infarct dementia commonly have a history of hypertension or cerebrovascular disease (fits, 'faints', transient ischaemic attacks or even cerebrovascular accidents). There may be other evidence of vascular disease, such as a history of ischaemic heart disease or carotid bruits or retinal vascular changes on examination. Focal neurological deficits may also be present. There is no evidence of a genetic component in the aetiology of this syndrome. Multi-infarct dementia is more common in men than in women.

Unlike the insidious onset and slowly progressive course of SDAT, multi-infarct dementia commonly has an acute onset (coinciding with an episode of infarction) and a step-wise course which reflects subsequent infarcts. Such acute events are often accompanied by episodes of acute brain syndrome and also by focal neurological deficits. In some cases, repeated episodes of acute brain syndrome are the only conspicuous manifestation of this process.

The pattern of cognitive deficits in mult-infarct dementia tends to be more patchy than in SDAT and there is also characteristically better preservation of the personality. Some patients display emotional lability, which can sometimes be so marked as to suggest an affective disorder. However, emotions are characteristically very shallow, appearing facile. The patient appears to 'switch off' his crying just as quickly as it began, and crying and laughter may closely follow each other. This pattern of emotional response is different from that seen in affective disorders. It is important to remember, however, that episodes of depression may also occur, particularly in the early stages of dementia while that patient's insight is still relatively preserved.

Although there are clear distinctions between multi-infarct and Alzheimer-type dementia in aetiology and pathogenesis, the two conditions frequently coexist, resulting in a clinical picture which combines elements of both presentations. FTTTT

Reversible causes of dementia include:

A. hypothyroidism
B. normal pressure hydrocephalus
C. neurosyphilis
D. Pick's disease
E. subdural haematoma

In most cases, dementia is caused by progressive and irreversible degenerative processes. However, it is particularly important in all cases to exclude other causes of this syndrome which may be reversible with appropriate treatment, or at least allow deterioration to be arrested. There are many such treatable causes of dementia, including depressive pseudodementia ★, anaemia, endocrine abnormalities (such as hypothyroidism, parathyroid disorders and Cushing's syndrome), vitamin deficiencies (such as deficiencies of B12, folate and thiamine), metabolic imbalance (such as renal or hepatic failure), infections (like neurosyphilis and cerebral tuberculosis), space-occupying lesions (such as subdural haematomata or tumours), normal-pressure hydrocephalus, etc. The extent to which such reversible causes of dementia are pursued will depend on the nature and presentation of each individual case (see MCQ 27).

Clinical features suggestive of normal pressure hydrocephalus include shuffling ataxic gait, psychomotor retardation and the early development of incontinence, in addition to features of dementia. This condition accounts for about 7% of cases of dementia starting over the age of 65 years. The cause is reduced resorption of cerebrospinal fluid by the arachnoid villi. This is commonly due to previous damage to the arachnoid mater, due to subarachnoid haemorrhage or meningitis, for example. The cerebrospinal fluid pressure, and flow within the ventricular system, are both normal but the ventricles are enlarged. Cortical sulci and gyri are relatively unaffected. Treatment is usually by ventriculo-peritoneal shunt. Some doubt has been cast on the risk-benefit ratio of this procedure and repeated cerebrospinal fluid removal has been suggested as an alternative to surgery.

The possibility of a subdural haematoma may be suggested by a history of head injury. As with other space-occupying lesions leading to dementia, intracranial pressure is usually raised and focal neurological signs may be present. The diagnosis is confirmed by computerised tomography of the brain.

Classical signs of neurosyphilis include optic atrophy and Argyll-Robertson pupils. Other focal signs including those of associated tabes dorsalis may be present. A wide variety of mental symptoms may be present. Adequate treatment is important to halt the progression of the disease and this may in some cases lead to an improvement in the symptoms, even those due to organic causes. Features suggesting of hypothyroidism include the characteristic appearance with thick, pale, dry skin and sparse hair. Cold intolerance may be present and clinical examination may reveal bradycardia and delayed relaxation of tendon reflexes.

Pick's disease, like Alzheimer's disease, is a progressive degenerative disorder of the brain for which there is no specific treatment. It is much less common than Alzheimer's disease. It gives rise to the syndrome of dementia but pathology is largely confined to the frontal and temporal lobes. Early signs of the disorder often include changes in personality and social behaviour without marked impairment of general intellect and memory. TTTFT

MCQ 21

The management of an elderly person with dementia:

A. is assisted by an initial domiciliary visit
B. always requires acute hospital admission
C. may involve techniques of reality orientation
D. does not involve supportive psychotherapy
E. should never include the administration of ECT

In Britain, less than 4% of people over the age of 65 live in institutions of some sort (psychogeriatric units, long-stay geriatric wards, old people's homes). Estimates of the prevalence of dementia vary, but at least 5% of people over 65 have mild dementia and a further 5% suffer from severe dementia. Most of these are supported in the community.

Visiting the patient at home is very valuable in making a thorough assessment, particularly if dementia is suspected. In addition to physical and mental state examination, it is possible to gauge how the person functions on a day-to-day basis. The home setting offers useful clues regarding adequacy of domestic skills, nutrition and personal hygiene which could not be elicited in a clinical setting. For the patient also, an assessment at home usually less disruptive and distressing, and allows some measure of the patient's optimal level of functioning. In addition, help may be sought from neighbours, friends and relatives in obtaining a more detailed history. Home visits also allow an assessment of the local resources available to help to support the patient— How willing are neighbours to become involved? Can the person continue to find his way to the corner shop next door? And so on. To maintain the individual in the community, local resources need to be mobilised and coordinated. These may include home helps, meals-on-wheels, day centres, church and other voluntary organisations. For those people who can cope with living in the community but cannot any longer be entirely independent, sheltered accommodation is a possibility.

Removing the person from his home environment (for admission to hospital or even outpatient assessment) may cause increased confusion and bewilderment and may exacerbate an already present acute brain syndrome. Having spent some time away from home, it may be difficult for the person to settle back into the home environment. However, there are circumstances in which hospital admission is necessary, such as in a medical emergency, when further investigations are judged necessary which cannot be done at home, or when cognitive and/or physical deterioration has become too advanced to allow the person to remain at home safely.

The diagnosis of dementia carries with it potentially devastating implications for both the patient and his family. In the early stages, when insight is preserved, patient and family will benefit from continued advice, explanation, understanding and support (supportive psychotherapy). In later stages the focus of this work moves to the immediate family who generally bear the burden of caring for the patient on a day-to-day basis.

Structured programmes of activity and stimulation help to combat sensory deprivation which may exacerbate the dementing process. Psychological techniques may be useful which are designed to encourage the individual to make optimal use of his remaining mental resources. Of these techniques, the most commonly used is reality orientation, in which the person's orientation in time and place, and his knowledge and understanding of his surroundings, are reinforced by repeated and clear cues. For example, some day centres and psychogeriatric wards have a large and conspicuous board listing information like 'Today's date is . . .', 'The next meal will be . . .', and all the rooms are clearly signposted.

Medical aspects of management should not be neglected. Apart from physical illnesses, which should be appropriately treated, demented people also develop other psychiatric disorders. These require appropriate treatment in their own right. Antidepressants, hypnotics or antipsychotic medications may be helpful. Dementia is not itself a contraindication for ECT, which may be beneficial in the management of severe or resistant depression. However, care should be taken to exclude conditions overrepresented among those with dementia which are contraindications for ECT, such as raised intracranial pressure, space-occupying lesions, recent stroke or myocardial infarct and neurosyphilis. TFTFF

Concerning psychiatric disorders in the elderly (more than 65 years old):

A. The prevalence of dementia in the age group over 65 years is 10–20%
B. functional psychiatric disorders constitute the most frequent diagnostic group
C. depression, particularly when severe, is commonly resistant to treatment
D. paranoid psychoses are commonly symptomatic of organic brain syndromes
E. benign senescent forgetfulness is a common prelude to dementia

Among those over 65 years old, the overall prevalence of psychiatric illness rises with age, due to a steep increase with age in incidence of dementia. Among those in their late 60's and early 70's, organic disorders as a whole account for approximately half the cases of psychiatric disorder. This proportion reaches more than nine in ten cases among those over 85 years old. The prevalence of dementia is approximately 10–20%, although figures vary considerably from one study to another depending on the degree of cognitive impairment necessary to classify someone as demented, and also other factors. A problem sometimes encountered in research and also in clinical practice is to distinguish between the ordinary effects of ageing and very mild dementia. Dementia is not just qualitatively different from normal ageing, but also qualitively different, as indicated by its distinct pathology (MCQ 18). Impairment of memory and decreasing mental agility are of course common with ageing, and to distinguish these from dementia, some specialists favour the use of the term **benign senescent forgetfulness**. This is not a prelude to dementia, but a normal part of the process of ageing.

The diagnosis of functional psychiatric disorders (see MCQ 2) in the elderly is often complicated by the fact that they occur along with acute or chronic brain syndromes—depressive pseudodementia ★ is a good example. Paranoid states may be part of an organic psychosis, but may also occur in the absence of any conspicuous brain pathology, where they commonly involve delusions which may be very elaborate and systematised. For example, someone suffering such a state is able to produce very complex explanations of how his persecutors gain access to his home to interfere with his food. Hallucinations may also be present, but the personality is often very well preserved, as social functioning may be. Such paranoid states, arising for the first time after the age of 50 years, are sometimes termed **(late) paraphrenia**. They are associated with impaired hearing and other sensory deficits, and patients commonly lack any previous history of psychiatric disturbance. Paraphrenia is uncommon—it has a low prevalence in the community, and accounts for only 5–10% of psychiatric admissions in the age group of over 65 years. However, its recognition is important, as it may be very distressing to the sufferer and often responds to treatment with antipsychotic drugs.

In some cases, the presentation of psychiatric disturbance in later life represents the continuation of chronic or recurrent functional psychiatric disorders which began when the person was younger. Thus a further diagnosis to consider in an elderly patient with a paranoid psychosis is a longstanding schizophrenic disorder.

Functional disorders among the elderly, whether or not they coexist with brain syndromes, should be treated as they are in younger people, but bearing in mind that the elderly may show greater sensitivity to the adverse effects of drugs and may require smaller doses. In general, there is no reason to expect a poorer response to appropriate treatments among the elderly than among younger patients. TFFTF

MCQ 23

People with epilepsy:

A. have a lower mean general intelligence than the general population
B. are no more prone to depression than the general population
C. are overrepresented in the prison population
D. have a higher suicide rate than the general population
E. have psychiatric disorders whose symptoms can usually be predicted on the basis of the underlying brain pathology

The associations between epilepsy and psychiatric disorder are complex and influenced by numerous factors. These include the effects of the fits themselves (and of the treatments used to control them), effects due to any underlying brain damage predisposing to epilepsy and also the effects of having a chronic illness.

Brain damage which may give rise to epilepsy may also cause cognitive impairment. Thus a proportion of epileptics show lower than average intelligence. Besides the direct influence of brain damage, the assessment of intelligence is influenced by the effects of the fits themselves and also the medication used to treat them. However, in terms of aetiology the most common type of epilepsy is idiopathic epilepsy, in which there is no evidence of conspicuous brain damage. Epileptics as a group follow the same distribution curve of intelligence as does the population as a whole.

In both adults and children with epilepsy, the prevalence of psychiatric disorder is two to four times greater than in control populations. The nature of this morbidity cannot be solely accounted for by the nature of associated brain damage which in many cases may not be in evidence. Psychosocial effects such as parental attitudes of overprotection or rejection, the disruption of schooling, play and work, and the stigmatising effects of the condition, also play an important role. The most common psychiatric diagnosis is of depression. The prevalence of both deliberate self-harm and of suicide is higher among epileptics than in the general population.

Epileptics are overrepresented in the prison population and comprise some 7–8 per 1000 inmates. However, the relationship between epilepsy and crime is complex. Episodes of automatic behaviour of which the individual is unaware (**automatisms**) do occur as a component of seizures experienced by some epileptics. While criminal behaviour during an automatism does occur, this is a rare phenomenon. Although associated personality disorder and psychiatric illness may explain the link between epilepsy and crime in some cases, it is probable that the overrepresentation of epileptics in prisons represents the operation of common adverse biological and psychosocial influences such as poor health care and subcultural violence. FFTTF

In temporal lobe epilepsy:

A. the prevalence of psychiatric morbidity is higher than in other forms of epilepsy
B. the precise symptoms of the fits are quite likely to alter from one seizure to the next
C. complex auras involving several sensory modalities are less common than in seizures arising from occipital lobe foci
D. the prodrome is characteristically shorter than the aura (if there is one)
E. routine electroencephalography reveals characteristic abnormalities in almost all cases

Focal seizures originate more commonly in the temporal lobes than in any other part of the brain. The most common pathology underlying temporal lobe foci is mesial temporal sclerosis, produced by anoxia (such as occurs in some prolonged febrile convulsions in childhood). The temporal lobes are also vulnerable to damage during head injury. Temporal lobe foci may also be due to tumours, vascular lesions or hamartomas.

As with other types of epilepsy, temporal lobe fits may be preceded by a **prodrome**, a time when the epileptic may feel uncomfortable, irritable or restless, which acts as a type of warning of an impending seizure. Prodromes have a gradual onset and may last hours, even days in some cases. By contrast, the **aura** begins abruptly and is brief (seconds to minutes). The aura is really part of the seizure itself, and its symptoms suggest the site in the brain of the epileptic focus. The temporal lobes are unique within the brain for the complexity of the auras they produce. Epileptic foci elsewhere produce auras comprising simple motor or sensory phenomena. By contrast, temporal lobe auras may be very complex and may involve several sensory modalities (vision, smell, touch, etc.). Temporal lobe auras may involve autonomic, perceptual, affective and cognitive components. Such states may be mistaken for a variety of psychiatric disorders, such as panic attacks or brief psychotic episodes. Such psychiatric disturbance is described as **ictal** when it forms part of the seizure. Such ictal phenomena must be distinguished from **post-ictal** disorders, which are always preceded by a fit and follow immediately after a fit, and **inter-ictal** disorders, which occur between seizures. Overall, there is a higher prevalence of psychiatric disorders associated with temporal lobe epilepsy than with other forms of epilepsy. Some researchers have described an inter-ictal behavioural syndrome of temporal lobe epilepsy, which includes features like excessive or unusual religious and philosophical interests, low sexual interest and obsessionality. How prevalent this syndrome is, and whether it is specific to temporal lobe epileptics, as is claimed, remains controversial.

It is characteristic of epileptic seizures that, no matter how complex their symptoms, they follow the same pattern from one fit to the next. This is because the ictal features are determined by the precise focus of the seizure. Although the fits will share common features, which come together in a specific sequence, some fits will not progress as far as others, and here some of the expected symptoms of the fit may be absent. Similarly, some focal seizures will lead on to a generalised convulsion (secondary generalisation) while others will not. Some people have more than one focus, and may then experience correspondingly greater numbers of seizure types. However, if the pattern of an individual's fits is markedly changeable, this suggests that they are not due to epilepsy but are **pseudoepileptic seizures** (also termed pseudoseizures), which represent a form of hysterical conversion ★.

Electroencephalography is often helpful in confirming the diagnosis. However, the routine inter-ictal EEG (or even the post-ictal EEG) may show no abnormalities suggestive of an epileptic focus and more detailed tests are required (such as a sleep EEG or an EEG using special sphenoidal leads). TFFFF

The following are virtually diagnostic of epileptic seizures but occur only exceptionally if at all in pseudoepileptic fits:

A. a raised serum prolactin after the fit
B. biting one's tongue or other self-injury
C. status epilepticus
D. fits lasting as long as twenty minutes
E. an extensor plantar reflex

The diagnosis of epilepsy has profound implications for the patient and his family. These include the consequences of long-term medication and the impact of seizures on employment, driving and many other aspects of living. It is thus particularly important to distinguish epilepsy from other clinical syndromes resembling it, notably pseudoepileptic seizures. The distinction is often complicated by the coexistence of both types of fit in the same individual. Also, many people who are found to have pseudoepileptic seizures have a history of epilepsy in the past.

As with other forms of hysterical conversion ★, clues may be found by careful attention to the presenting problem—in this case, the details of the seizures. Consecutive epileptic seizures in one individual always follow a similar pattern, while pseudoepileptic fits may not do so (MCQ 24). Epileptic seizures do not last more than a few minutes (unless there are serial seizures or the person goes into status epilepticus). Thus a story of fits lasting half an hour on each occasion leads to the suspicion of pseudoepileptic fits. Episodes of 'status' have been reported with pseudoepileptic seizures, thus status itself cannot be used to distinguish the two syndromes. People having pseudo-seizures may injure themselves, may be incontinent and may even show signs of impaired consciousness (such as lack of response to painful stimuli). However, upgoing plantars which become flexer after the seizure are indicative of epilepsy. Post-ictally, someone with epilepsy invariably feels worse than before; some people with pseudoepileptic seizures report feeling better after their seizures. Some people with pseudoepileptic seizures only have fits in particular situations, notably when other people are present. This can sometimes help to distinguish these fits from epileptic seizures. However, epileptic fits can sometimes be induced by specific circumstances or even be self-induced.

An abnormal ictal or post-ictal EEG may help in diagnosis, but such an EEG is less helpful if it shows no particular abnormalities (MCQ 27). Serum prolactin levels are commonly considerably raised following epileptic seizures, but not after pseudoepileptic fits. Thus a blood sample for prolactin levels 20 minutes after a fit may be useful. TFFFT

MCQ 26

Following head injury:

A. the length of retrograde amnesia is a better predictor of brain damage than the length of anterograde (post-traumatic) amnesia
B. location of the brain damage seldom determines the nature of the cognitive or other psychiatric problems
C. diffuse brain damage is less common with injuries which penetrate the skull than with non-penetrating injuries
D. the post-traumatic syndrome is more likely after severe head injuries than after relatively minor ones
E. personality changes are almost always transient

The relationship between head injury and subsequent cognitive and other psychiatric disturbances is complex. Important factors include the nature, location and severity of the head injury, subsequent organic problems (such as focal neurological deficits and epilepsy), the emotional impact of the injury and the patient's premorbid personality.

Penetrating injuries (involving skull fractures) are likely to produce local damage adjacent to the site of the injury. Non-penetrating injuries tend to give more diffuse damage. Clinically, the severity of such diffuse brain damage is related to the length of post-traumatic amnesia. This is defined as the time from the moment of injury to the time of resumption of normal continuous memory. As an approximate guide, a period of post-traumatic amnesia of longer than 24 hours usually results in significant brain damage, while this is less likely with shorter post-traumatic amnesic gaps. The period of retrograde amnesia (the time from the injury back to the last clear memory the patient can recall before the injury) tends to be much shorter than the post-traumatic gap and is less useful as an indicator of brain damage.

In general, most psychiatric problems after head injury are directly related in their severity to the degree of brain damage. One exception to this is the **post-traumatic (post-concussional) syndrome**. This is characterised by headaches and dizziness, together with other symptoms like insomnia, irritability and forgetfulness. These symptoms may be incapacitating. The basis of the syndrome remains controversial (some question even whether this condition exists as a clear syndrome). Some studies have reported that the condition is more common after mild head injuries than after severe ones.

The site of any brain damage may affect the type of psychiatric disturbance which follows the injury. For example, schizophrenia-like psychoses are more common after damage to the temporal lobes than any other parts of the brain. Frontal lobe damage can give rise to the **frontal lobe syndrome**, characterised by impulsive behaviour, disinhibition (including sexual and aggressive) and shallow mood. The patient often comes across as immature, self-centred and socially inappropriate.

Among other important factors which influence psychiatric morbidity after head injury, premorbid personality is important. Personality changes after head injury sometimes reflect an exaggeration of existing personality traits, although this is not always the case. Personality changes are usually persistent and may be dramatic. There is some evidence that particular personality traits may themselves predispose to head injury, although this has not been well established. FTTFF

Procedures which may be useful in excluding organic causes of psychiatric disorders include:

A. physical examination
B. electroencephalography
C. therapeutic trail of antipsychotic medication
D. cognitive testing
E. urine drug screening

All patients require complete physical examination when they first present. Whether or not the examination reveals any abnormalities is not itself helpful—the presence of abnormalities does not necessarily indicate an organic aetiology, neither is this excluded by the absence of abnormalities. However, specific signs may be found of possible intracranial or extracranial causes of organic states—focal neurological deficits are an example of the former.

Similarly, all patients presenting with psychiatric symptoms should be given a brief cognitive assessment, comprising at least tests of orientation, attention and concentration, recent memory and general knowledge. If these reveal abnormalities, or there is evidence from the history to suggest an organic cause to the disturbance, more detailed cognitive examination is necessary.

An EEG without significant abnormalities virtually excludes the diagnosis of acute brain syndrome, and the EEG in the chronic brain syndromes also commonly shows abnormalities. Note, however, that while a normal EEG may be helpful in this context, an abnormal recording is less so. Some individuals may have an abnormal EEG quite independently of the aetiology of their psychiatric disturbance.

Urine analysis may reveal the presence of abused drugs—a specimen should be collected from patients presenting with psychotic symptoms who are suspected of taking illicit drugs. This investigation has the limitation that most abused drugs (and their metabolites) can only be traced in the urine for a short time after they have been taken. The main exception to this is cannabis, which can be detected in the urine for quite long periods.

Having decided that a particular psychiatric presentation is likely to have an organic aetiology, the next step is to investigate its cause. The extent to which this is pursued will depend on the details of each individual case. However, an initial screening battery would appropriately include haemoglobin and full blood count, urea and electrolytes, blood sugar and thyroid function tests, together with chest X-ray. The result of these tests might suggest further appropriate investigations.

Therapeutic trials of medication are sometimes necessary in psychiatry as elsewhere in medicine (for example, a pyrexia of unknown aetiology may be managed with a trial of anti-tuberculosis drugs). However, no psychotropic drug is sufficiently specific in its actions to allow response to treatment to give accurate information about the diagnosis. For example, most psychotropic drugs are sedative to some extent, and may help someone suffering from an anxiety state—if the drug used is an antipsychotic, this does not imply that the patient is or was psychotic. In the organic psychoses, psychotropic medication is used for the management of symptoms rather than the underlying cause(s), and care must be taken to avoid the symptomatic treatment masking the important signs of the cause of the disorder. For example, heavy sedation might make it more difficult to recognise the evolution of an intra-cranial bleed. TTFTT.

Schizophrenia

MCQ 28

Which of following statements about schizophrenia are true?

A. lack of insight occurs during at least some phases of the illness
B. disturbance of mood is uncommon in schizophrenia
C. in many cases, the disorder begins early in adult life
D. the disorder can begin with an insidious deterioration of occupational and social function
E. it is rare for substantial impairment of social and occupational function to persist after delusions and hallucinations have resolved

Schizophrenia is a psychosis in which a wide variety of disturbances of thought, mood, perception and behaviour can occur. As in other psychotic illnesses, lack of insight and distortions of reality occur in at least some phases of the illness. There is no single symptom or group of symptoms unique to schizophrenia, though certain types of delusions and hallucinations, designated by Schneider as **first-rank symptoms** ★ of schizophrenia, are regarded as strong evidence of schizophrenia in certain circumstances. Perhaps the most characteristic feature that distinguishes schizophrenia from other illnesses is incongruity between thought, emotion and behaviour. Thus, for example, a schizophrenic patient may receive bad news with little sign of emotion, or describe in vivid detail how his persecutors are torturing him without appearing afraid. Bleuler introduced the name 'schizophrenia' to denote the fragmentation of the various aspects of psychological function which occurs in this illness. Unfortunately, attributes such as incongruity are difficult to assess reliably.

Another characteristic that contributes to the concept of schizophrenia, but is of only limited use in making the diagnosis, is the tendency for the illness to run a chronic course, with persisting occupational and social handicap. Kraepelin, who described the illness before Bleuler and gave it the name 'dementia praecox', regarded a chronic course as one of the cardinal characteristics which distinguished this disorder from manic-depressive psychosis. However, illnesses which present with symptoms typical of schizophrenia can follow various different courses over time, ranging from complete remission after one episode, to persistence of severe symptoms throughout adult life. Most psychiatrists do not use the term schizophrenia to describe very brief psychotic illnesses. For example, the American diagnostic manual DSM-IIIR ★ specifies, arbitrarily, that the illness must persist for at least six months to justify use of the diagnosis schizophrenia. Illnesses of shorter duration, but with similar symptoms, are described as **schizophreniform**.

In some cases which run a chronic course, florid symptoms such as delusions and hallucinations persist throughout the illness, but more commonly chronic schizophrenic patients exhibit transient episodes of florid symptoms superimposed on persisting disorganisation or impoverishment of thought and emotion. Although less dramatic, this persistent disorganisation or impoverishment of thought and emotion can result in marked occupational and social handicap.

Typically schizophrenia presents in early adult life, sometimes beginning suddenly, but in other cases developing insidiously, with a gradual deterioration of social and occupational function. Schizophrenia beginning in later adult life tends to be different. In cases with later onset, delusions are usually prominent but more circumscribed, and there is less widespread disintegration of mental life (see MCQ 34). However, these differences are a matter of degree. TFTTF

MCQ 29

Regarding the epidemiology of schizophrenia:

A. the life-time risk of suffering from schizophrenia is estimated at 0.85%
B. schizophrenia is much less common in Africa than in Europe
C. the prevalence of schizophrenia is higher in rural areas than in urban areas
D. the age of onset of schizophrenia tends to be later in females than in males
E. schizophrenic patients are more likely to have been born in winter than in summer

Studies in many different parts of the world have demonstrated a relatively uniform incidence of schizophrenia. The life-time risk of suffering from schizophrenia is approximately 0.85%. There are several small regions, such as the west of Ireland, northern Sweden and part of Yugoslavia, where the risk is higher. Despite the relative uniformity, on a global scale, of the occurrence of schizophrenia, within any one country the prevalence of schizophrenia is higher in urban areas than in rural ones. This probably reflects a tendency for schizophrenic patients who have difficulty adapting socially to drift into cities.

The life-time risk of suffering from schizophrenia is approximately the same for males and for females. However, the onset tends to be earlier in males. The peak of onset is in the third decade for males and in the fourth decade for females.

Several studies have shown that schizophrenic patients are more likely to have been born in the winter months than in the summer months. Although the studies carried out in the southern hemisphere have been less extensive, this pattern appears to occur in both hemispheres. It raises the possibility that an environmental factor acting in the perinatal period can play a role in the aetiology of schizophrenia. TFFTT

There is good evidence that the following make a significant contribution to the aetiology of schizophrenia:

A. prolonged separation from mother during infancy
B. genetic factors
C. parental communication which places an adolescent in a 'double bind'
D. unemployment
E. foods containing gluten

The aetiology of schizophrenia remains unknown. There is much evidence that a variety of organic and social factors can play a role in determining the onset and/or course of the illness. The most firmly established aetiological factor is genetic. The concordance for schizophrenia among monozygotic twins is about 50%, while the concordance among dizygotic twins is about 12% (MCQ 10). Despite the much higher concordance among monozygotic twins, the fact that the concordance among individuals with identical genes is not 100% demonstrates that other factors must play a role. For example, perinatal brain injury has been implicated. There is good evidence that psychosocial factors, such as stressful life events, can precipitate episodes of acute disturbance in schizophrenia, but there is no substantial evidence that psychosocial factors can produce the illness in an individual who does not have a special suscepti-bility. In particular, despite wide interest in the hypothesis that inappropriate parental communication during adolescence plays a causal role in schizophre-nia, the available evidence does not support such a hypothesis. Similarly, there is no evidence that separation from mother during infancy plays a causal role in schizophrenia.

The evidence that stressful life events can precipitate episodes of acute disturbance in schizophrenia provides reason to suppose that unemployment could precipitate an acute episode, but there is no direct evidence that unemployment plays a substantial causal role. It has been proposed that various dietary factors, including foods containing gluten, cause schizophrenia, but adequate evidence for such proposals is lacking. FTFFF

Regarding the genetics of schizophrenia:

A. a schizophrenic patient should be strongly advised against having children because of the risk that the children will develop schizophrenia
B. the child of a schizophrenic woman is much less likely to develop schizophrenia if adopted into a normal family in infancy
C. the gene for schizophrenia is a Mendelian recessive gene
D. there is an increased prevalence of alcohol abuse among the relatives of schizophrenic patients
E. the schizophrenic illness is usually more severe and persistent in schizophrenic patients who have a family history of affective disorder

The risk that a child who has one schizophrenic parent will develop schizophrenia is about 12%, compared with a life-time risk of 0.85% in the general population (MCQ 29). A schizophrenic patient considering whether or not to have children should be told of this moderate risk, but in itself this risk does not constitute adequate reason for stongly advising against having children. For the patient, there is also a risk that the stresses of pregnancy and parenthood will exacerbate the illness. All these factors need to be discussed with the patient and his or her spouse, to allow them to make a decision based on adequate information.

Research studies have found that, for children of schizophrenic women, the risk of the child itself developing schizophrenia is no different if the child is raised by its natural parents or adopted into a normal family in infancy. On the other hand, a child of a normal mother adopted into a family with a schizophrenic parent does not suffer an increased risk of developing schizophrenia (MCQ 10).

The mode of inheritance of the susceptibility to schizophrenia remains unknown. The graduation of risk between first-, second- and higher degree relatives is not consistent with inheritance via a Mendelian recessive gene, but is consistent with polygenic inheritance.

There is evidence of an increased risk of some other types of psychiatric illness among the relatives of schizophrenic patients. For example, the prevalence of alcohol abuse is higher than expected. Such observations are consistent with the concept that schizophrenia is part of a spectrum of diseases, but this concept is a subject of debate. There is also evidence that genetic factors related to affective disorder influence the nature of schizophrenia. Schizophrenic patients with a family history of affective illness are less likely to suffer a severe, persistent schizophrenic illness than schizophrenic patients without a family history of affective disorder. FFFTF

The following statements are correct regarding the neuropathology and neurochemistry of schizophrenia:

A. many post-mortem studies have found non-specific abnormalities in the brains of schizophrenic patients
B. some schizophrenic patients have enlarged cerebral ventricles
C. virus-like particles are commonly observed in the hippocampus in patients with schizophrenia
D. it is well established that a defect in metabolism in schizophrenic patients leads to the accumulation of abnormal metabolites which are hallucinogenic
E. there is evidence that schizophrenia involves underactivity of dopamine in certain parts of the brain

Post-mortem examination of the brains of schizophrenic patients has revealed a wide variety of abnormalities. These include evidence of dysplasia of the frontal lobes, decreased volume of limbic structures and basal ganglia, and evidence of degeneration in the mid-brain and brain stem. However, no specific abnormality has been identified which is characteristic of schizophrenia. Further non-specific evidence of structural abnormalities of the brain in schizophrenia is provided by the evidence from X-ray computed tomography that some schizophrenic patients have enlarged cerebral ventricles.

The similarity between the chemical structure of some hallucinogenic drugs and catecholamine neurotransmitters has prompted the hypothesis that abnormal metabolites of catecholamine neurotransmitters might occur in schizophrenia. This hypothesis received further support from the finding of abnormal catecholamine metabolites in the urine of schizophrenic patients. However, it appears that this finding was an artifact arising from the atypical diet of schizophrenic patients. Thus, there is no convincing evidence favouring the hypothesis that abnormal catecholamine metabolites play a role in schizophrenia.

The observations that dopamine blocking agents relieve some of the symptoms of schizophrenia, and that dopamine agonist drugs can exacerbate schizophrenic symptoms, suggest that dopamine overactivity plays a role in the genesis of schizophrenic symptoms. Also, some post-mortem studies of the brains of schizophrenic patients have found an increased number of dopamine receptors in certain deep nuclei, such as the caudate nucleus. While this finding might be an artifact induced by previous treatment with dopamine blocking drugs, recent evidence from studies of dopamine receptor numbers in the caudate nucleus of living patients indicates that the increased number of receptors is present prior to treatment. To date, this finding has been inconsistent, but, if replicated to future research studies, it would constitute substantial evidence that dopamine overactivity occurs in schizophrenia.

Virus-like particles have been reported in the cerebrospinal fluid of schizophrenic patients, but the significance of these particles remains unknown. In combination with other observations, such as the increased proportion of winter births among schizophrenic patients, this evidence supports the proposal that viruses could play a role in the transmission of schizophrenia. However, there is little direct evidence for the viral theory of schizophrenia. TTFFF

The following are characteristic of schizophrenia:

A. third person auditory hallucinations
B. bizarre behaviour accompanying a gradual but profound decline in occupational and social function
C. the belief that alien thoughts are inserted into one's mind
D. a feeling of necessity to ruminate on an idea, which is resisted by the patient
E. marked flattening of affect

There are no symptoms which are pathognomonic of schizophrenia. Nonetheless, it is customary in clinical practice to pay particular attention to the presence of certain delusions and hallucinations known as **Schneiderian first-rank symptoms**. The presence of these, in the absence of any other organic brain disease, are considered strong grounds for making a diagnosis of schizophrenia. The first-rank symptoms include primary delusions ★, passivity phenomena and certain types of auditory hallucinations. Passivity phenomena include delusions of control, such as the belief that one's will is taken over by an alien influence, and certain delusions concerning the possession of thought, such as thought insertion ★ and thought broadcast ★. The two types of auditory hallucination classed as Schneiderian first-rank symptoms are hallucinatory voices talking about oneself in the third person and hearing one's thoughts spoken aloud (**thought echo**).

While the majority of schizophrenic patients do suffer from Schneiderian first-rank symptoms at some time during their illness, there are some who do not. There are other symptoms which also suggest a diagnosis of schizophrenia. These include marked flatness of affect, incongruity of affect, and certain types of formal thought disorder ★. Bizarre behaviour accompanied by a gradual but profound decline in occupational and social function is also typical of schizophrenia. Such features are much more difficult to assess reliably than the first-rank symptoms but, when accompanied by serious and persistent impairment of occupational and social function, support a diagnosis of schizophrenia, even in the absence of first-rank symptoms.

A feeling of necessity to ruminate on a particular idea, despite the attempts by the patient to resist the rumination, is characteristic of obsessional neurosis ★. Although schizophrenic patients sometimes suffer from obsessional neuroses, such a neurotic symptom cannot be regarded as characteristic of schizophrenia. TTTFT

Concerning sub-types or sub-syndromes of schizophrenia:

A. the traditional classification of schizophrenia into the sub-types paranoid, hebephrenic, catatonic and simple schizophrenia is unsatisfactory because individual cases often have a mixture of the characteristics of these sub-types
B. non-paranoid schizophrenic patients have a better prognosis than paranoid schizophrenics
C. positive and negative symptoms of schizophrenia are mutually exclusive
D. chronic schizophrenic patients are more likely than acute schizophrenic patients to exhibit evidence of neurological dysfunction
E. schizophrenic patients with a family history of schizophrenia are more likely to exhibit evidence of structural brain damage than those without a family history of schizophrenia.

Because schizophrenia is a very heterogeneous disorder, there have been attempts to sub-divide it into various types. The traditional types are paranoid, hebephrenic, catatonic and simple. **Paranoid schizophrenia** is characterised by delusions and hallucinations with relatively good preservation of personality. **Hebephrenia** tends to have an earlier onset and is characterised by 'silly' speech, emotion and behaviour (incongruity of behaviour and affect, formal thought disorder, etc.). In **catatonic schizophrenia**, abnormal movements and postures are a prominent feature. These include waxy flexibility (in which the patient allows himself to be placed into an uncomfortable or awkward posture which he is then able to maintain for long periods), ambitendence (where the patient begins one movement then moves the opposite way) and 'mitgehen' (the patient moves a limb in response to slight pressure from the examiner despite being told to keep the limb still). **Simple schizophrenia** consists of an insidious deterioration of personality, with a paucity of florid features. However, the majority of cases exhibit features of several of these different types of illness, making sub-typing difficult and often futile.

Despite the difficulties with attempts to subdivide schizophrenia, the striking differences between cases in the extent to which personality attributes are impaired, has led to several different dichotomous classifications. One such dichotomy is the distinction between paranoid and non-paranoid schizophrenia. Characteristically, paranoid schizophrenia has a relatively late onset, and the clinical presentation is dominated by delusions, while personality is relatively well preserved. Many paranoid schizophrenic patients are able to maintain interpersonal relationships and sustain a reasonable work record. In contrast non-paranoid cases tend to suffer from disorganisation or impoverishment of their thinking and emotions, leading to insidious deterioration of occupational and social function. Thus there is a tendency for non-paranoid patients to be more seriously handicapped by their illness. Nonetheless, the distinction between paranoid and non-paranoid illnesses is not clear-cut, and it is not unknown for patients with paranoid schizophrenia to become seriously disabled.

Another dichotomous classification in schizophrenia is based on the distribution between positive and negative symptoms. **Positive symptoms** (and signs) reflect the presence of an abnormal mental function. Delusions, hallucinations and incoherent speech are examples of positive symptoms. **Negative symptoms** (and signs) reflect the absence or diminution of a mental function which is present in normal individuals. Poverty of speech and flatness of affect are examples (strictly speaking, these observable attributes should be called negative signs, but it is customary to refer to them as symptoms). Positive symptoms tend to occur together and thus constitute a syndrome. Similarly, negative symptoms tend to occur together and constitute a negative syndrome which can be distinguished from the positive syndrome. However, the positive and negative syndromes are not mutually exclusive and in many instances positive and negative syndromes coexist in an individual patient.

Yet another dichotomy is the distinction between acute and chronic schizophrenia. Chronic schizophrenic patients tend to exhibit a somewhat different symptom profile, and in particular are more likely to have flatness of affect. In addition chronic schizophrenic patients show many similarities to patients with known brain damage.

Despite their differing conceptual bases, the dichotomies above overlap with each other. Chronic schizophrenia, non-paranoid schizophrenia and the negative syndrome share features in common. Similarly, acute schizophrenia, paranoid schizophrenia and the positive syndrome share common attributes. The fact that attempts to subdivide schizophrenia have led to the delineation of these similar but nonetheless different dichotomies indicates that schizophrenia is not an amorphous aggregate of disparate signs and symptoms, but even so, it has proved difficult to identify a clear-cut segregation of attributes of the illness into syndromes or sub-types.

Another approach to the classification of schizophrenia is to attempt to delineate differences in aetiology. It has long been recognised that many brain diseases can produce a schizophrenia-like illness, but these secondary schizophrenia-like illnesses have been considered to be quite distinct from 'primary' schizophrenia. As evidence has accumulated indicating a variety of relatively subtle abnormalities of structure and function of the brains of schizophrenic patients, the distinction between 'primary' schizophrenia and secondary schizophrenia-like illnesses has become more arbitrary.

The observation that schizophrenic patients with a family history of schizophrenia are less likely to exhibit evidence of structural brain damage has led to the proposal that familial and non-familial schizophrenia are two distinct types of illness. However, an alternative interpretation of this observation is that various factors including genetic endowment and history of brain damage contribute in a cumulative manner to susceptibility to schizophrenia. If this were so, cases with a genetic predisposition to schizophrenia would be expected to require a lesser contribution from brain trauma, to exceed a threshold beyond which the manifestation of schizophrenia would be inevitable. According to this viewpoint, the distinction between familial and non-familial cases is not a distinction of major importance. TFFTF

The following symptoms are of value in distinguishing between schizophrenia and affective psychoses:

A. hallucinatory voices calling the patient by name
B. delusions of persecution
C. incongruent affect
D. a delusional belief in possessing a special identity
E. the experience that one's actions are under alien control

The distinction between schizophrenia and affective psychosis is often difficult, as any of the symptoms of affective psychosis can occur in schizophrenia, and conversely, symptoms typical of schizophrenia such as Schneiderian first-rank symptoms can occur in affective psychosis. Nonetheless, despite the overlap in clinical presentation, it is important to make the distinction between schizophrenia and affective psychosis because they tend to follow different temporal courses and require different forms of management.

In general, incongruity between affect and content of thought suggests a diagnosis of schizophrenia, whereas mood-congruent delusions and hallucinations are suggestive of affective psychosis (MCQ 45). Thus, inappropriate affect is more typical of schizophrenia. The experience that one's actions are under alien control is quite uncommon in affective psychosis, but is a first-rank symptom of schizophrenia and therefore suggests a diagnosis of schizophrenia. Hallucinatory voices calling the patient by name occur quite commonly in both schizophrenia and in affective psychosis, and in themselves are of little value in distinguishing between the two diagnoses, though the degree of congruence between the hallucinatory experience and mood does help in making the distinction. Delusions of persecution can occur in psychotic illnesses of any type, and are therefore of little use in distinguishing between different psychoses. A delusional belief in possessing a special identity suggests either mania or schizophrenia, and in itself is of limited value in distinguishing the two illnesses. A delusional belief in possessing a grandiose identity, accompanied by an elated mood, would support a diagnosis of mania.

In addition to assessment of current symptoms, information concerning family psychiatric history and an account of the patient's past episodes of illness countribute to making the diagnostic distinction between schizophrenia and affective psychosis. FFTFT.

Regarding mood disturbance in schizophrenia:

A. many schizophrenic patients have a significant depression of mood at some time during their illness
B. antipsychotic medication usually exacerbates depressed mood in schizophrenic patients
C. tricyclic antidepressants have consistently been shown to be of value in treating depressed mood in schizophrenia
D. most cases of depressed mood in schizophrenia appear to arise as a psychological reaction to awareness of the handicaps of schizophrenia
E. apathy in schizophrenic patients is usually associated with depressed mood

Depression is common is schizophrenia, and can occur during the prodromal phase preceding acute episodes of schizophrenic symptoms, during the acute episode itself, and during relatively stable periods between acute episodes. About 20% of acutely disturbed schizophrenic patients have depressed mood, and about 10% of randomly selected chronic patients have depressed mood at the time of assessment. It is probable that the majority of schizophrenic patients suffer from significantly depressed mood at some time during their schizophrenic illness.

It has been suggested that antipsychotic medication might cause depressed mood in schizophrenic patients, but systematic studies have demonstrated that depressed mood often resolves in parallel with schizophrenic symptoms after antipsychotic treatment begins, suggesting that in such cases the antipsychotic medication helps relieve the depression. Recent research suggests that tricyclic antidepressants may be effective in treating depression in schizophrenic patients, although previous studies have consistently reported no benefit from tricyclics in such patients. There is thus very limited evidence that tricyclic antidepressants may be of value in treating depression in schizophrenics.

It has been suggested that depression is schizophrenic patients is a psychological response to awareness of the problems of suffering from schizophrenia. The observation that depression can occur at an early phase in a schizophrenic illness, and in some cases actually precedes the development of psychotic symptoms, demonstrates that such a psychological response cannot account for all cases of depression in schizophrenia, and the balance of evidence suggests that in the majority of cases, depression in schizophrenia is an intrinsic part of the schizophrenic illness. Nonetheless, in the management of schizophrenic patients it is important to be sensitive to the patient's psychological response to his illness.

Apathy is a common problem in chronic schizophrenia. In the majority of cases it is not accompanied by depression. TFFFF

The following statements are true regarding intellectual and neurological function in schizophrenia:

A. a substantial number of chronic schizophrenic patients show evidence of intellectual impairment
B. intellectual impairment is associated with poor outcome in schizophrenia
C. in schizophrenia, poor performance on tests of abstract reasoning is strongly associated with having delusions
D. in schizophrenic patients, there is a higher prevalence of impaired motor coordination and impaired higher sensory functions such as astereognosis than in the general population
E. abnormal involuntary movements were not reported in schizophrenia prior to the introduction of antipsychotic medication in the 1950's

In some schizophrenic patients, there may be evidence of a variety of signs of brain dysfunction, including poor performance on tests of intellectual function, impairment of motor coordination and higher sensory functions, and abnormal involuntary movements.

The links between such signs of brain dysfunction and schizophrenia have been the subject of considerable debate. According to one view, brain dysfunction is an intrinsic part of the schizophrenic illness in some cases. Alternatively, it could be attributable to factors related to treatment, such as poor motivation, unstimulating institutional environment or side-effects of antipsychotic medication. At present, the balance of evidence favours the first view, that brain dysfunction is part of the schizophrenic illness. For example, some studies have found a correlation between intellectual impairment and brain ventricular enlargement. Furthermore, the majority of studies find no correlation between amount or duration of antipsychotic medication, and intellectual or neurological impairment.

Significant intellectual impairment is usually associated with chronic symptoms and signs, such as poverty of speech and flatness of affect. Patients who suffer acute schizophrenic illness, with florid symptoms such as delusions and hallucinations but without persistent poverty of speech and flatness of affect, are much less likely to show evidence of intellectual impairment. Intellectual impairment is often associated with a poor outcome. However, it is unusual for the intellectual impairment to take the form of a progressive dementia. The severity of intellectual impairment is not strongly related to the duration of illness.

Various forms of abnormal involuntary movements, including choreiform movements of face and limbs, were reported in schizophrenic patients long before antipsychotic medication was introduced. Since the introduction of antipsychotic medication such abnormal movements have been reported to be much more common, and the term **tardive dyskinesia** ★ has been introduced to describe them. At present it is uncertain to what extent abnormal involuntary movements in schizophrenic patients reflect the brain's response to medication, but it is probable that factors related to the illness itself play a role in determining susceptibility to exhibit abnormal involuntary movements. TTFTF

The following factors are associated with relapse in schizophrenia:

A. stimulating life events, which may be either positive or negative
B. regular contact for several hours daily with a caring parent who is over-protective
C. critical comments by parents
D. a diet rich in cheese and/or red wine
E. discontinuation of antipsychotic medication after all delusions and hallu-cinations have resolved

Although the nature of schizophrenia remains an enigma, a number of well-replicated studies have provided firm guidance for managing schizophrenia in a way that reduces the risk of relapse. It has been demonstrated that relapse can be precipitated by stimulating life events ★. Therefore, patients should be helped to organise their lives in a way that minimises the occurrence of stressful events. Furthermore, relapse is more likely if the patient has regular contact with relatives who are emotionally over-involved with the patient or over-protective, or who are hostile or make critical comments about the patient. Such relatives are said to display **high expressed emotion**. Reducing the level of expressed emotion in such families through counselling results in a lower rate of relapse. In some cases, patients may be helped by decreasing the amount of their contact with relatives who are too critical or over-involved. However, it is important to remember that not all families are over-involved or excessively critical and even when they are, in many instances the family has more potential for good than for harm. For patients who have a limited ability to make new relationships, family members might be the only source of sustained support apart from that provided by professional services.

Antipsychotic medication plays an important part in reducing the frequency of relapse in schizophrenia. Even after acute symptoms have resolved, regular treatment with antipsychotic drugs should be maintained because relapse rate is much higher in those who discontinue medication.

There is little evidence to suggest that particular foods precipitate relapse in schizophrenia. However, medication prescribed for other conditions can occasionally produce psychosis, and therefore might precipitate relapse of schizophrenia. In particular, L-dopa prescribed as treatment for Parkinson's disease can exacerbate psychotic symptoms. Abused drugs, especially amphe-tamine, can precipitate schizophrenic relapse. There is also some evidence that cannabis precipitates psychotic episodes in predisposed individuals, and it is possible that schizophrenic patients are at special risk. TTTFT

In the treatment of acute schizophrenia:

A. alleviation of stress by psychosocial means makes only a minor contribution to the management of the acute episodes

B. it is usually better to use an antipsychotic drug which has antipsychotic action but minimal sedative action, rather than one with both antipsychotic and sedative action

C. In those cases where antipsychotic medication achieves a substantial antipsychotic effect, the major part of this effect is achieved within the first three days of treatment

D. negative symptoms such as flattened affect are usually more responsive to antipsychotic treatment than are positive symptoms such as delusions

E. ECT produces a more sustained benefit in schizophrenia than antipsychotic medication

An important part of the management of acute schizophrenia is modification of the patient's environment so as to minimise stress. In many instances this is achieved by admitting the patient to hospital. Often the relief of pressure together with the supportive environment of a hospital ward produce a substantial improvement in the patient's mental state within a few days. In principle, it is possible to relieve stress and provide support without admission to hospital, but in the majority of cases such management in the community can only be achieved by a dedicated, adequately staffed community care team.

Antipsychotic medication is also important. Often patients suffering from an acute schizophrenic episode are restless and it is best to use an antipsychotic drug such as chlorpromazine, which has sedative action in addition to antipsychotic action (MCQ 122). The sedative effects of antipsychotic medication are usually achieved quite rapidly, but the antipsychotic action produces a more gradual effect, which often is not clearly discernible until the second week of treatment. In the majority of cases antipsychotic medication alleviates positive symptoms such as delusions and hallucinations, but the effect on negative symptoms such as flatness of affect is less clear-cut.

ECT is no more effective than antipsychotic medication in the treatment of acute schizophrenia, and its beneficial effect is rarely sustained, so it is therefore only rarely used to treat schizophrenia. It has been claimed that ECT is especially effective in the treatment of catatonia, but whether or not this effectiveness can be attributed to the fact that in some cases of catatonia there is a marked affective disturbance, remains a subject of debate. FFFFF

In the long-term management of schizophrenia:

A. antipsychotic medication should be discontinued when the patient has been free of psychotic symptoms for six months
B. gradual resumption of an active lifestyle should be encouraged when an episode of acute schizophrenic disturbance has resolved
C. lack of social stimulation is likely to contribute to deterioration in social function in schizophrenic patients
D. attempts to modify emotional interactions in the family have negligible influence on the course of schizophrenia
E. individual psychotherapy based on psychodynamic principles is of proven value in schizophrenia

There is good evidence from many studies that discontinuation of antipsychotic medication substantially increases the risk of relapse in the following two years. However, many questions concerning the relative benefits and risks of long-term prophylactic antipsychotic treatment remain unanswered. There are no clear guidelines for identifying the minority of cases who would not suffer a relapse even if medication were to be discontinued. Secondly, there is little reliable evidence to help answer the question of whether or not prophylactic medication should be continued indefinitely. The very few long-term studies that have been conducted indicate that several decades after the initial episode, a substantial proportion of schizophrenic patients can lead a stable life without taking medication. Unfortunately, it is extremely difficult to conduct sound scientific studies of treatment over such long periods of time. It is currently accepted practice to offer long-term prophylactic antipsychotic treatment.

Satisfactory long-term prophylaxis against schizophrenic relapse depends on achieving reliable administration of an adequate dose of antipsychotic medication, while minimising debilitating side-effects. It is usually preferable to choose a drug with relatively little sedative effect. For this reason, chlorpromazine is not generally suitable for long-term prophylactic use. It is often appropriate to administer maintenance antipsychotic medication in the form of depot injections, in which the medication is suspended in a oil from which it is released slowly. Typically, injections at three-week intervals maintain a sufficiently steady plasma drug level. Depot injections are useful for those patients who find difficulty in taking oral medication regularly.

Psychosocial interventions are as important as pharmacological treatments in helping schizophrenic patients to avoid unnecessary handicap. Research has demonstrated that those patients subjected to a stultifying environment suffer much greater handicap than patients whose environment is more favourable and less institutionalised. However, it is also the case that vigorous attempts to stimulate the patients increase the frequency of schizophrenic relapse. It is therefore important to encourage the gradual resumption of autonomy and activity when an episode of acute schizophrenic disturbance has resolved. The patient should be encouraged to resume as active a lifestyle as possible via a series of carefully graded steps, but strong pressure should be avoided.

Close contact with a relative who is emotionally over-involved, or who expresses critical comments, increases the likelihood of schizophrenic relapse

(MCQ 38). However, it has been demonstrated that informing relatives about the nature of schizophrenia, and helping them find constructive ways of solving problems within the family, produces a lower relapse rate.

The majority of schizophrenic patients need some form of psychosocial support, which can be provided by the professional mental health workers and by relatives and friends. There is no evidence that psychodynamic psychotherapy is helpful in schizophrenia, and there is a risk that the psychological stress generated by some forms of psychotherapy might be harmful to schizophrenic patients. FTTFF

MCQ 41

Regarding the provision of services for schizophrenic patients:

A. schizophrenic patients with persistent delusions should generally be offered long-term inpatient care in hospital

B. long-term hospital care is the major cause of apathy in schizophrenic patients

C. schizophrenic patients should generally be discouraged from living with their families

D. for a substantial number of chronic schizophrenic patients, a house shared with other patients, with supervision by a community psychiatric nurse, is an appropriate form of accommodation

E. there is good evidence that the occupational needs of most chronic schizophrenic patients are best catered for by brief training courses rather than longer-term sheltered work

A small proportion of schizophrenic patients suffer persistent delusions and hallucinations despite treatment with antipsychotic medication. Provided that such persistent symptoms do not lead the patient to act in a way that is likely to harm himself or others, persistent delusions or hallucinations are not in themselves an adequate reason for long-term hospital inpatient care. However, some chronic schizophrenic patients do require sustained support if they are to avoid drifting into a derelict state. In many cases, apathy and disorganisation of activity are the major factors in such a social deterioration. It is probable that the majority of schizophrenic patients could receive the level of long-term support which they require from well-organised community psychiatric services, but adequate resources and energetic work by the community care staff are necessary to prevent schizophrenic patients living in the community being forced to lead impoverished, lonely lives.

For those patients who cannot cope with the stress of living independently, some form of supportive accommodation is essential. For those who have families able to care for them, the family home may provide the best option, at least during the early years of adult life. Although close contact with over-involved or critical relatives can promote relapse, appropriate education and support for the family is often a better option than separation from the family. Nonetheless, in some circumstances, the strain suffered by families with a severely disturbed schizophrenic member is too great, and accommodation away from the family is desirable. A house shared with other patients, with necessary support provided by psychiatric nursing staff, is suitable in many cases. The degree of support provided by the nursing staff can vary according to need, ranging from regular visits by a community psychiatric nurse, to more intensive support from resident nursing staff.

For the small proportion of schizophrenic patients who are persistently too disturbed to allow them to settle into a household, long-term hospital care might be the best option. An asylum can provide the intensive nursing and a range of supervised occupations needed by severely disturbed patients.

Schizophrenia reduces the abilities of many patients to work. Several factors contribute to this difficulty. Impairment of concentration is very common in schizophrenia, and often persists after acute symptoms have resolved. Many schizophrenic patients become very distressed when under pressure. In addition, apathy is a serious problem in some cases. In the past, apathy in schizophrenic patients was attributed to the effects of a stultifying institutional environment, but it appears more likely to be an intrinsic part of the illness. For many chronic schizophrenic patients relatively long-term sheltered work is appropriate. Studies of improvement of work performance of schizophrenic patients usually show a slow linear increase in performance, rather than a rapid initial rise followed by a plateau characteristic of normal learning. Therefore, short-term training courses are often of little benefit to chronic schizophrenic patients. FFFTF

Affective Disorders

MCQ 42

Symptoms common to all types of depression are:

A. loss of self-esteem
B. increased risk of suicide
C. constantly low, unchanging mood
D. insomnia
E. loss of interest in everyday events

Lowering of mood is characteristically the main symptom of depression. The depressed person feels sad, miserable and blue, and may feel tearful or actually cry frequently. For some patients, this low mood varies with their circumstances—there may be some situations in which an individual hardly feels depressed at all. However, for others, the low mood becomes completely unvarying and does not lift even when something pleasant happens. This unchanging low mood is characteristic of **endogenous depression**, otherwise called **melancholia** ★ (as 'endogenous depression' is a confusing term—see MCQ 44—this type of depression will be referred to throughout this book as 'melancholia'). In extreme cases, patients may say that they are unable to cry or even to experience any feelings.

All depressed patients have lowered self-esteem. They feel worthless and inherently bad—at worst, such feelings may be accompanied by delusions that the patient must die because of his sins or worthlessness. Depression of all kinds increases the risk of suicide, probably via the feelings of hopelessness and helplessness, and because of the low self-esteem. The majority of completed suicides are preceded by depression (MCQ 88).

Most depressed patients lose interest and the ability to take pleasure in their usual activities, and lose some of their ability to concentrate. In melancholia this may be total—nothing in life is able to give pleasure or to excite interest.

A number of 'biological' or 'vegetative' symptoms ★ occur in melancholia which are not characteristic of other types of depresion. The commonest of these is insomnia—which may be difficulty getting to sleep, disturbed nights or early waking, or a mixture of all three. Not all patients with depression show these features—about 10% have over-sleeping and fatigue. Loss of appetite and loss of weight can occur but again a small proportion show increase of these functions. Loss of interest in sex, lowered libido and, in females, menstrual disturbance occur in melancholia. Headaches, heavy feelings in the abdomen and constipation are all frequent accompaniments of melancholia. Psychomotor symptoms like retardation (slowed movements) or agitation (restlessness, pacing, hand-wringing) occur in severe forms of melancholia but are not features of other types of depression. Other symptoms which occur only in some forms of depression are delusions and hallucinations, which are found in psychotic depression ★. TTFFT

The following symptoms are recognised to be features of 'endogenous' depression (melancholia) rather than other types of depression:

A. diurnal variation in mood—worse in the morning
B. total loss of interest and pleasure in usual activities
C. difficulty falling asleep
D. loss of appetite
E. loss of concentration

Melancholia ('endogenous' depression) is a clinical syndrome whose main symptom is profound lowering of mood unreactive to events going on around the patient. The patient's mood does not lift, even in response to something good happening. This total inability to take interest in or derive pleasure from customary activities is termed **anhedonia**.

Melancholia is usually associated with several 'biological' or 'vegetative' symptoms ★. Among these are loss of appetite and loss of weight which are sometimes severe and can even endanger life. Insomnia is common. The characteristic pattern involves waking in the early hours of the morning rather than difficulty falling asleep (that is, *terminal* rather than *initial* insomnia). Sometimes the patient wakes as early as 2.00 a.m., unable to get back to sleep. Also associated with melancholia is a diurnal pattern of mood—mood is at its lowest on wakening and improves during the day. Note that other types of depression may also show apparently diurnal variations in mood, but here mood tends to be responsive to regular events in the person's life, like a spouse coming home, or feeling lonely on arriving home to an empty flat after a day's work. Psychomotor disturbances like retardation or agitation may be present (MCQ 42).

Although concentration is often impaired in melancholia, this also occurs in other forms of depression (MCQ 42). Anxiety (nervousness, tenseness, jumpiness) may be present but is much more often a feature of neurotic depression ★ than melancholia.

Melancholia may also be differentiated from other types of depression by its usual course, which tends to involve discrete episodes, each with the same features as the last, with a return to normal function between episodes. By contrast, neurotic depression ★ comes and goes but often the patients do not function well between episodes. TTFTF

Regarding the classification of depression and other affective disorders:

A. the presence or absence of biological symptoms is an important feature in classifying a depressive disorder
B. in most cases, the term 'unipolar affective disorder' refers to a disorder with recurrent episodes of mania
C. bipolar affective disorder involves episodes of depression and, at other times, episodes of mania
D. patients with neurotic depression commonly have episodes of mania at other times in their lives
E. 'endogenous' depression is less often precipitated by severe life events than other forms of depression

Several classifications of depression are available, but none is entirely satisfactory. Of all the types of depression, melancholia or 'endogenous' depression ★ is the most adequately defined. The main feature distinguishing melancholia from other types of depression is the presence of 'biological' symptoms ★. Previously, it was believed that this type of depression arose 'from within', independently of life events or personal circumstances—hence the term 'endogenous'. This form of depression was contrasted with 'reactive' depression, which was considered to follow adverse life events. However, it is clear from research that the 'endogenous' pattern of depression (involving biological symptoms) is preceded by severe life events just as frequently as is the 'reactive' type of depression. More recently, 'endogenous' has been used purely as a short-hand way of describing depression with biological features, without necessarily involving any assumptions about possible precipitants. However, this use of 'endogenous' remains confusing, the main reason why some psychiatrists now prefer to use the term 'melancholia', which will be adopted in place of endogenous depression throughout this book.

Another common classification divides depression into 'psychotic' and 'neurotic' forms. Strictly speaking, the term 'psychotic' should be reserved for depression with delusions and/or hallucinations, the content or theme of which (poverty, guilt, illness, etc.) fit in with mood. By contrast, 'neurotic' depression is a mixture of many ill-defined but generally mild to moderate mood disorders, involving other neurotic symptoms like anxiety, hypochondriasis or agoraphobia. The failure of this classification lies in the fact that some types of depression (notably melancholia) are neither neurotic nor necessarily psychotic.

A suitable starting point for a clinically useful classification of depression is the presence or absence of biological features, since these have implications for treatment (MCQ 51). Depression which lacks biological features may be called **non-endogenous**. If, in addition, other neurotic features are present, such as hypochondriasis, this becomes **neurotic** depression. When biological symptoms are present, this is **endogenous** depression (**melancholia**). If, in addition, there are mood-congruent delusions and/or hallucinations, **psychotic** depression may be diagnosed. Psychotic depression can be seen as a subtype of melancholia—it is unusual for psychotic symptoms to be present in a depression when there are no biological features. Melancholia and psychotic depression can be further subdivided according to past history. Where someone who has melancholia or psychotic depression has a past history of mania, this is classified as **bipolar affective disorder**. If there is a history of episodes of melancholia but no episodes of mania (or vice versa), this is termed **unipolar affective disorder**. In practice, this last term is usually confined to cases of recurrent depression—recurrent mania with no episodes of depression is rare. This subdivision into unipolar and bipolar disorders does not encompass neurotic and other non-endogenous types of depression—these have no particular associations with mania. Unipolar and bipolar affective disorders together comprise **manic-depressive disorder**. Note that, while neurotic symptoms may be present in some cases of melancholia, the converse is not true—if biological symptoms are present, even when neurotic symptoms may be prominent, this is classified as melancholia (see the symptom hierarchy—MCQ 2).

Although depressed mood is a prominent feature in most cases of depression, whatever the type, depression may sometimes present with little evidence of lowered mood and other symptoms (particularly somatic ones) predominating. This is termed **masked depression** ★ TFTFF

MCQ 45

Which of the following types of hallucination are characteristic of psychotic depression?

A. third person auditory hallucinations
B. voices commenting on the patient's actions
C. voices saying derogatory things about the patient
D. voices telling the patient to commit suicide
E. voices echoing the patient's thoughts

Psychotic phenomena (delusions or hallucinations), to be characteristic of depression, must be mood-congruent, that is, they can be seen as a consequence of severely abnormal mood (see MCQ 35). Third person auditory hallucinations, voices commenting on the patient's actions and voices echoing the patient's thoughts do not necessarily have any particular mood or feeling associated with them. Such hallucinations are often associated with blunted affect and are more likely to be found in schizophrenia than in affective disorder. By contrast, voices making derogatory comments about the patient or telling him to commit suicide can be seen as a psychotic extension of a depressed mood and so are characteristic of psychotic depression.

The same rule applies to delusions. If these are congruent with mood (such as delusions of worthlessness, guilt, poverty or bodily illness), they are indicative of psychotic depression rather than schizophrenia.

In mania also, delusions and hallucinations are commonly mood-congruent. Manic patients are often expansive in their mood and thought and have grandiose delusions, for example that they have special powers. Delusions other than grandiose may also be congruent with mood—for example, someone who is manic and believes that his special powers must be used to catch criminals might develop persecutory delusions about the police when his attempts to assist them are rebuffed.

This rule, regarding the congruence with mood of psychotic phenomena in affective disorder, while clinically useful, is only a rule of thumb and does not always apply. There are no truly pathognomonic symptoms of affective disorder. FFTTF

In mania, the patient:

A. often has a labile mood with bouts of crying
B. is always euphoric
C. is almost always psychotic
D. sometimes has first-rank symptoms of schizophrenia
E. often has formal thought disorder

While the hallmark of the manic state is an infectious optimism and euphoria, this is by no means always present. Many manic patients are hostile and aggressive during their illness and on taking a history from relatives this proves to be out of character for the patient. Mood is usually changeable. Euphoria and grandiosity, when thwarted, may give way to irritability or aggression and quite often to tearfulness.

40—50% of manic patients have psychotic symptoms. The delusions are usually grandiose or paranoid, and hallucinations, which occur in 10% of all manic patients, are always auditory. Schneiderian first-rank symptoms ★, although more a feature of schizophrenia than affective disorder, occur in approximately one in eight cases of mania.

The type of formal thought disorder which is characteristic of mania is **flight of ideas** ★. This is often accompanied by **pressure of speech**. TFFTT

MCQ 47

Which of the following are characteristic of mania?

A. increased risk-taking
B. hypochondriasis
C. sexual disinhibition
D. sleep disturbance
E. overactivity

Hypochondriasis is the only symptom listed which is uncharacteristic of hypomania. The manic patient usually has a sense of general well-being and neither looks nor feels ill, although transient hypochondriacal complaints do sometimes occur.

Sleep is commonly disturbed, and insomnia or early morning waking can be an early sign of a manic episode. Patients with mania are invariably hyperactive, although this is rarely productive or focused. During a manic illness, patients tend to be boastful and conceited, and easily irritated if others fail to cooperate with their plans. Their grandiose ideas regarding an inflated sense of their personal importance can become delusional. Sexual interest and activity are increased, and patients are commonly disinhibited in company, passing personal remarks, often with sexual innuendo.

Delusional beliefs in their special abilities or powers may lead manic patients to behave in a reckless fashion. This clearly has important implications in management, as such behaviour may put the patient's life at risk. TFTTT

Recognised features of neurotic depression include:

A. paranoid delusions
B. depersonalisation
C. anxiety
D. suicide attempts
E. agoraphobia

The diagnoses of melancholia and psychotic depression are based on the presence of particular symptoms (MCQ 43). By contrast, the main distinguishing feature of neurotic depression is the **absence** of the biological symptoms of depression. The term 'neurotic depression' covers a range of rather different conditions. For both these reasons, it is better to avoid simply classifying a person's illness as a neurotic depression and instead think in terms of a more detailed formulation, including a description of the symptoms, the history of the illness (which may be chronic) and the precipitants.

So-called neurotic depression may involve a variety of neurotic symptoms. Anxiety is very common, and may be the predominant feature. Phobic states (notably agoraphobia ★) and depersonalisation ★ may also occur.

The presence of paranoid delusions indicates a diagnosis of psychotic depression, paranoid schizophrenia ★ or other paranoid state.

Attempts at suicide (or other episodes of deliberate self-harm) are commoner in all forms of depression than in the general population. Such episodes are not restricted to patients with melancholia. Remember, however, that many attempts at deliberate self-harm occur in the absence of any symptoms of depression, in the context of an acute interpersonal trauma, like a row with a boyfriend (MCQ 89). FTTTT

MCQ 49

Regarding the epidemiology of the affective disorders:

A. the point prevalence of depressive symptoms in the general population is approximately 15%
B. both unipolar and bipolar affective disorder have a lower prevalence in married people compared with those who are single
C. the incidence of affective disorder tends to rise with age
D. it has been established that endocrine and genetic factors largely account for the differences between men and women in prevalence of unipolar affective disorder
E. the incidence of depression in women is not substantially raised following the menopause

Symptoms of depression are common in the general population, with a point prevalence of 13–20%. Affective *disorder* is much less common. The overall prevalence of unipolar affective disorder is approximately 3% in males, and 4–9% in females. Bipolar affective disorder has a lower prevalence, more approximately equal between the sexes.

In unipolar affective disorder, factors other than sex associated with increased prevalence rates include being unmarried (especially being divorced or separated), lower socioeconomic class and younger age. The difference in prevalence between the sexes is complex and cannot be accounted for by one or two factors alone. The increased incidence of depression in the six months following childbirth (MCQ 115) suggests the importance of endocrine factors, although their influence is complex. However, the menopause is not associated with a rise in the incidence of depression. Many other factors are likely to be relevant, such as the observation that women are more likely than men to talk openly about symptoms of depression with their friends and to present with these symptoms to their general practitioner. The relative contribution of each of these factors has yet to be adequately established.

The risk factors for bipolar affective disorder are somewhat different. Not only is the prevalence similar in both sexes, but there is no clear association with marital or socioeconomic status. In common with unipolar affective disorder, there is a higher incidence of bipolar affective disorder in the younger age groups. Bipolar affective disorder tends to have an earlier onset (characteristically in the late 20's) compared with unipolar affective disorder (which commonly begins in the fourth decade). TFFFT

Recognised aetiological factors in affective disorder include:

A. lack of confiding relationship
B. a positive family history of affective disorder
C. lack of paid employment
D. significant life events which would commonly be regarded as positive, like a family wedding
E. use of propranolol to control hypertension

It is evident from family, twin and adoption studies (MCQ 10) that there is a genetic contribution to the affective disorders. This is more significant in bipolar than in unipolar affective disorder. Other biological factors which contribute to the aetiology of depression include a wide range of illnesses ranging from infections (such as infectious mononucleosis) to neoplasms and endocrine disorders such as hypothyroidism, hyperparathyroidism and Cushing's disease. In addition, some commonly prescribed drugs may precipitate depression. These include propranolol, methyldopa, L-dopa, oral contraceptives and sulphonamides. However, such drugs seldom precipitate depression in the absence of other aetiological factors, notably a past history of affective disorder or a positive family history. Remember also that the illnesses these drugs are intended to treat may themselves also contribute to the onset of depression.

People who develop affective disorders have commonly experienced an excess of significant life events shortly before the onset of their disorder. Although these life events commonly involve losses, it is difficult to generalise. The meaning of any given life event must be understood in the context of the person experiencing it (see MCQ 11). An event like a family wedding, which would seem positive and pleasurable to many people, may for the parents of a single child represent the break-up of their family more than anything else. Not everyone responds to adverse life events, even the most serious ones, by becoming depressed. This has led to the suggestion that there are particular factors which make some people more vulnerable than others to develop depression in response to adverse life events. For example, in one study of urban women, adverse life events were more likely to lead to depression if there was no confiding relationship with a husband or partner, if the woman had no employment outside the home and if there were several young children at home. In practice, it is difficult to make a clear distinction between the influence of such vulnerability factors and the life events themselves. TTTTT

In the treatment of depression and other affective disorders:

A. all types of depression are equally likely to respond to treatment with tricyclic antidepressants
B. it is useful to distinguish between the treatment of the acute illness and longer-term prophylaxis
C. psychotherapy may be hazardous in bipolar affective disorder
D. depression which has been precipitated by a life event is less likely to respond to physical treatments (antidepressants or ECT) than depression which has no clearly evident precipitants
E. neurotic depression responds less favourably to drug treatments than melancholia

The presence of biological symptoms is associated with a greater likelihood of a favourable response to physical treatments (antidepressants or ECT). Thus melancholia and psychotic depression are more likely than 'neurotic' depression to respond to tricyclic antidepressants. This is the case regardless of the presence or absence of any clear precipitants for the depressive episode; these do not influence the likely response to treatment. However, this does not mean that aetiology should be ignored. For example, if an episode of depression is thought to have arisen from an accumulation of personal difficulties, the acute episode may respond to drug treatments, but returning the individual to the same adverse environment is likely to make him or her vulnerable to further depressive episodes. A family history of affective disorder also predicts a favourable response to physical treatments.

Although neurotic depression is less likely than melancholia to respond to drug treatments, the use of physical treatments is not precluded. In particular, there is some evidence that monoamine oxidase inhibitors are effective in cases of neurotic depression. Indeed, some psychiatrists advocate neurotic or other 'non-endogenous' types of depression as the main indications for the use of monoamine oxidase inhibitors.

It is useful to distinguish in terms of treatment between the acute episode of affective disorder and longer-term prophylaxis. For melancholia or psychotic depression, acute treatment involves adequate therapeutic doses of antidepressants ★ or ECT ★. Smaller doses of antidepressants may be used for prophylaxis. In bipolar affective disorder, the risk of further episodes is even greater than in unipolar affective disorder, and prophylactic lithium ★ is often indicated. It may also be appropriate to address factors which maintain the individual's vulnerability to further episodes of depression, like marital conflict or an absence of social supports.

In general, psychotherapy has little part to play in the acute management of severe cases of affective disorder, although supportive psychotherapy is appropriate, for relatives as well as patients. In less severe cases, psychotherapy may play an important part in treatment. Cognitive therapy ★ in particular is being increasingly used and has been shown to be effective. However, use of other forms of psychotherapy involves greater caution. Exploratory psychotherapy may be appropriate in some cases of neurotic depression. However, this approach, if offered to someone with unipolar or bipolar affective disorder, may precipitate further episodes of illness (see MCQ 132). FTTFF

Which of the following represent an adequate trial of treatment in a case of melancholia (endogenous depression)?

A. amitriptyline 75 mg at night for 1 month
B. imipramine 150 mg at night for 1 week
C. 5 ECT treatments spread over 2 weeks
D. clomipramine 200 mg daily for 6 weeks
E. 15 ECT treatments spread over 5–6 weeks

With all antidepressants (given at adequate doses), there is inevitably a delay of at least 10–14 days before their antidepressant action becomes evident. This applies not only to the tricyclic antidepressants but others also, including monoamine oxidase inhibitors. This delay can be longer if the patient has been depressed for some time. Some cases of depression turn out to be 'resistant' to particular antidepressants, but no firm conclusions can be drawn regarding the efficacy of any treatment unless the antidepressant is given at therapeutic doses for a minimum of four weeks, and preferably six weeks.

With standard tricyclic antidepressants such as amitriptyline, imipramine and clomipramine, the *minimum* effective daily dose to treat an acute depressive episode is 100 mg. However, some patients fail to respond to this dose but do respond to higher doses. So unless the patient has been maintained for an adequate time on regular doses of at least 150 mg daily, no firm conclusion can be drawn regarding efficacy. Notice that these dosages only apply to the standard tricyclic antidepressants; newer antidepressants like mianserin, lofepramine, trazodone and fluvoxamine are used in different dosages. Patients vary considerably in their sensitivity not only to the antidepressant effects of the drugs but also the side-effects. In some cases, intolerance of side-effects may make it impossible to give adequate therapeutic doses of a given antidepressant. In such cases, another treatment needs to be chosen—either another antidepressant which does not produce the troublesome side-effect, or ECT. For some patients, it is possible and sometimes appropriate to increase the dose of their tricyclic antidepressant to 300 mg daily.

Unlike the antidepressant drugs, ECT can be very rapidly effective—there is no inevitable delay before treatment can be expected to take effect (MCQ 53). However, the response is not always immediate. An adequate trial of ECT requires at least six treatments. These are usually given twice or three times a week. If partial response has occurred after six treatments, then up to 15 treatments may be given, stopping when full remission is achieved. FFFTT

MCQ 53

Electroconvulsive therapy (ECT):

A. is ineffective for mood-congruent delusions of depression
B. is effective in all types of severe depression
C. acts by increasing noradrenaline levels in the amygdala
D. a course may consist of 10 or 12 treatments before full recovery
E. is a more hazardous procedure than a course of tricyclic antidepressants

ECT is a rapid and effective treatment for depressive illness with certain features. These are similar to the biological symptoms of depression—especially loss of appetite and weight, agitation and retardation. One well-conducted study showed that the most important feature indicating a good response to ECT in depression was the presence of depressive delusions and hallucinations (those with a content compatible with depressed mood, i.e. poverty, illness or guilt). Patients over 40 years old, and those with a family history of depression are more likely to respond. 'Neurotic' depression does not respond well to ECT, even though it may be severe.

Indications for ECT include failure to respond to appropriate antidepressant treatment at adequate therapeutic doses and severe depression requiring urgent treatment (with a high risk of suicide or in the presence of depressive stupor ★).

Improvement sometimes begins after the first treatment (see MCQ 52). Once remission has been achieved, there is no point in continuing with ECT. ECT has no prophylactic action (unlike antidepressant drugs, which may be continued for some time—usually at a smaller dose than that used to treat the acute episode—to minimise the risk of relapse).

Like many other effective treatments in medicine, the efficacy of ECT was first discovered by serendipity. Although its precise mechanism of action remains unknown, it is clear from research that the induction of seizure activity in the brain is essential for its efficacy.

The morbidity from side-effects and self-poisoning using tricyclics is greater than morbidity due to ECT, especially in the elderly. A recent survey reported a mortality rate due to ECT of 1 in 28 000 cases. This is far lower than the mortality due to depression itself. FFFTF

Lithium:

A. is used for prophylaxis of bipolar affective disorder
B. should be measured in plasma even when the patient has had a stable mood for a long time
C. plasma levels should be kept between 1.0 and 1.8 mmol/litre
D. may interact dangerously with diuretics
E. is prescribed in one dose at night because it is a sedative

The primary indication for lithium therapy is as prophylaxis to prevent further attacks of bipolar affective disorder ★. It is also used in the prophylaxis of unipolar affective disorder, but here it is not as effective as in bipolar affective disorder. It is sometimes used in combination with antipsychotic drugs in the acute treatment of mania.

Regular blood tests are an essential part of treatment with lithium. Because of the possible effects of lithium on the kidney and the thyroid, renal and thyroid function should be assessed before the start of treatment and then at regular intervals during treatment. If detected early, any abnormalities tend to be reversed on stopping the drug, or possibly only reducing the dose. However, as with all treatments, the possible costs must be carefully weighed against the likely benefits. For example, some patients with a history of severe and life-threatening episodes of affective illness who develop hypothyroidism while taking lithium prefer to continue on lithium and take thyroxine in addition rather than increase the risk of further episodes of mania or depression. Serum or plasma lithium levels should be measured at least once every three months as long as the patient takes the drug. This is to check the continuing stability of the drug's pharmacokinetics, as well as the patient's compliance. Plasma levels of 0.5–1.2 mmol/litre are adequate in acute treatment and should not be allowed to rise above 1.5 mmol/litre. Lower plasma levels are adequate for prophylaxis, although the minimum effective plasma level will vary from one patient to another. Many patients remain well with plasma levels of only 0.3 mmol/litre.

Unlike most of the antidepressants, lithium is not sedative. It may be prescribed as a single daily dose, but this is for the convenience of the patient and to encourage compliance. Some psychiatrists advocate using divided daily doses to avoid high peak concentrations and consequently minimise the risk of renal damage, but this remains controversial.

Lithium has important interactions with a number of other drugs. The commonest interaction involves sodium-losing diuretics—these cause lithium to be retained by the kidney, replacing sodium in the exchange mechanism in the distal tubule. This may lead to toxic plasma levels of lithium and consequently to severe adverse effects. TTFTF

The cognitive theory of depression:

A. states that depressed people are better able to recall unpleasant or sad memories than pleasant ones

B. states that non-depressed people are unduly optimistic in their appraisal of experiences and perceptions, while depressed people have more accurate cognitions

C. proposes that depressed patients show a characteristic way of thinking about themselves and the world

D. states that depression may be treated by the identification of cognitions ('automatic thoughts') and their counteraction by learning rational re-sponses

E. therapy based on the cognitive approach has been shown to be as effective as antidepressants in treating depression in outpatients and in general practice

The cognitive theory of depression holds that depression is associated with a group of maladaptive or unhelpful automatic thoughts (cognitions ★) which give rise to what Aaron Beck (a contemporary American psychiatrist and the leading exponent of cognitive therapy) has called the **negative cognitive triad**—a negative view of oneself, of the world and of the future. Depression involves negative and distorted cognitions, such as 'What's the point in trying? I'm bound to fail however hard I try.' The depressed person, like everyone else, usually takes for granted that his or her cognitions are true, even though he or she may not be fully aware of these automatic thoughts (see MCQ 134 for a further discussion of cognitive theory). Such negative cognitions make the depression worse, and vice versa, setting up a vicious circle. It has been suggested that, far from having abnormally negative cognitions, depressed people are more accurate in their automatic thoughts than others (those who are not depressed), who are unduly optimistic in their cognitions. Most cognitive therapists would disagree with this suggestion, which finds little support from existing research.

Cognitive therapy ★ aims to assist the patient to become more aware of and identify his abnormal cognitions and then to examine their validity, replacing them where necessary with reasoned responses. Thus in the example above, the patient may be asked to keep a record of his activities, rating each for the satisfaction and the pleasure they give him. Often, this technique can demons-trate that, far from being a total failure, and deriving no pleasure from anything, there are activities which give the patient pleasure as well as satisfaction. This serves as evidence against the original automatic thought, to which the patient is then able to make a rational response.

Several studies have now shown that, when properly carried out by trained therapists, cognitive therapy can be as effective as antidepressants in general practice or hospital outpatients. However, it is not useful in very severe or psychotic depression. There is also evidence that antidepressants and cognitive therapy together are more effective than each alone. Cognitive theory would predict that, if negative automatic thoughts play an important role in precipitating or maintaining depression, then cognitive therapy should have a prophylactic effect, minimising the likelihood of the patient being overcome by negative cognitions in the future. However, no evidence is yet available on this. FFTTT

The following symptoms are consistent with a typical grief reaction:

A. an initial period lasting about four months in which the bereaved person shows few if any signs of grief
B. delusional perception
C. hallucinations
D. somatic symptoms for which no organic cause can be found
E. signs of a return to one's previous ('normal') level of functioning within twelve months

Clinicians encounter many manifestations of loss among their patients—the death of loved ones, the loss of previously good health, the loss of part of the body, and so on. The process of grief is a natural and necessary response to significant losses such as these. The process involves the bereaved in several tasks which together form what has been described as 'grief work'. These tasks include a gradual acceptance of the reality of the loss, experiencing the pain of grief, severing some of the intense emotional ties with the lost person (or object) and readjustment by reinvesting emotional energy elsewhere and/or taking up different roles which are satisfying.

Several phases of grief can be recognised. Immediately following the loss, there is a period of shock or numbness and disbelief, lasting from a few hours to a few days. This is followed by 'acute grief', a phase of preoccupation with the lost person, of yearning and searching for him or her. The bereaved is likely to show many features of depression during this phase, which commonly reaches its peak within two weeks but may continue for some months. Episodes of crying, anxiety, anger, self-reproach and extreme fatigue are common. Other recognised features of this phase include somatic symptoms and hypochondriasis. There is often a sense of the lost person's presence, sometimes involving hearing his or her voice. However, delusional perception (a type of primary delusion ★) is not part of typical grief reaction—its presence points to the development of a psychiatric disorder. All these experiences, rather than being continual over a prolonged period, characteristically come in 'waves' of varying intensity. Gradually, after a few weeks or more, the bereaved takes the first steps towards readjustment to life without the deceased. The loved person can be remembered without evoking the previously intense emotions. Unwanted possessions of a dead spouse can be disposed of. Having previously withdrawn from friends and the outside world, the bereaved gradually begins to socialise more and to take renewed interest in the outside world. Signs of this are usually evident within the first twelve months of bereavement, although the final resolution of the grief process may take longer than this. Even then, the acute symptoms of grief may recur, for example on significant anniversaries (this is called an **anniversary reaction**).

Understanding the normal process of grief facilitates the recognition of abnormal or pathological grief, where the grief reaction is either delayed or distorted. FFTTT

The following are likely to be pathological one year after the death of a spouse:

A. prolonged depression (crying and sleep disturbance)
B. visual or auditory hallucinations of the spouse
C. loss of appetite and weight loss more than 2 kg
D. suicidal thoughts
E. feeling of worthlessness

Most bereaved people, although they find grief painful, manage to adjust to their loss. However, the process of grief may be distorted, delayed or displaced.

Sometimes, a bereaved person may find grief intolerably painful, and may then seek help. Here, helping the person to understand the process of grief and the necessity to complete the work of grief may be all that is necessary. It may be appropriate to 'legitimise' grief. For example, a person whose favourite pet has died may seek help because friends suggest that he could solve his pain by getting another pet; acknowledging that his dog was very important to him and that he needs to grieve its loss may allow him to tolerate his grief.

Grief may sometimes lead to clinical depression. The point at which normal feelings of sadness after losing a close relative become morbid depression is not exact and it is often difficult to decide when a normal grief reaction requires treatment with antidepressants and/or psychotherapy. However figures are available on the frequency with which individual 'symptoms' are manifest in the first year after bereavement: 33% of the bereaved still cry often after one year; 48% still have difficulty sleeping—so these features by themselves are not pathological; 16% of bereaved people have loss of appetite while 20% lose 2 kg or more in weight over a year. As with all other symptoms, these should only be interpreted in the context of the overall clinical picture. Appetite disturbance or weight loss as an isolated symptom is less likely to indicate a depressive disorder than when other features of depression are also present. Only 3% have suicidal thoughts and these should always be taken very seriously. Only 6% feel worthless after bereavement and this may indicate the likelihood of developing an abnormal bereavement reaction. 9% of bereaved people have hallucinations of the spouse one year after bereavement. They do not necessarily indicate depression and may be felt as comforting. However, if they are felt as distressing or even persecutory they may require treatment and then may be part of a psychotic depression brought on by the bereavement. Once again, this can only be decided by looking at the whole clinical picture.

Sometimes, bereaved people find the pain of grief too much to bear. Grief may then be **delayed** (in which case few if any of the typical features of grief will be present) or displaced. In **displaced grief**, the bereaved person may devote all his time and energy to some activity (which often has links with the person who died) to avoid confronting his grief. Neither delay nor displacement is by itself pathological—they are present to some degree in many grief reactions. Although delay and displacement are commonly present to some degree in typical grief reactions, it is when either is excessive that the grief process can be regarded as pathological. Excessive delay or displacement of grief is analogous to a phobic reaction, where the feared stimulus is the pain of grief. One way of managing such problems, analogous to desensitisation ★, is gradually to encourage the bereaved person to face the pain of grief and to undertake grief work. This is termed **guided mourning**. FFFTT

Neuroses

Neurotic symptoms:

A. are not caused by underlying organic brain disorder
B. are often accompanied by lack of insight
C. are common in patients attending their general practitioners
D. sometimes present in people who have no psychiatric disorder
E. may occur in schizophrenia

The term **neurosis** arose in the late eighteenth century to describe a disorder of the nervous system for which no organic cause could be found. Freud and the psychoanalytic school used the term **psychoneurosis** to denote a group of disorders with clear psychological causes, including hysteria, obsessional and anxiety disorders. Later German psychiatrists, including Jaspers and Schneider, thought of neuroses as reactions to stress occurring in people with abnormal personalities, and it is still useful to think of neurosis as a reaction of a particular kind of personality to stress.

ICD9 ★ defines neuroses as 'mental disorders without any demonstrable organic basis in which the patient may have considerable insight and has unimpaired reality testing, in that he does not confuse his morbid subjective experiences and fantasies with external reality. Behaviour may be greatly affected . . . but personality is not disorganised'. Neuroses often appear to be exaggerated forms of the normal reactions people have to stressful events. In other words, the difference between neurotic symptoms and everyday responses to stress may be quantitative rather than qualitative.

Individual neurotic symptoms are very common in the general population and may be evident in 80% of adults. On their own, such symptoms do not necessarily warrant a psychiatric diagnosis. It is difficult to define accurately the point at which such symptoms become severe enough and/or distressing enough to justify a psychiatric diagnosis. However, neurotic symptoms like anxiety, irritability, fatigue, insomnia and misery are common among patients presenting to general practitioners and may present together as an **undifferenti-ated neurosis**. Other common neurotic symptoms include hypochondriasis and other somatic complaints (without any physical basis). Obsessions and phobias may also be found.

Besides the undifferentiated neuroses, specific neurotic syndromes occur in which there are particular combinations of symptoms. Such syndromes include the anxiety neuroses ★, hysteria ★ and obsessional states ★.

Neurotic symptoms commonly occur in other psychiatric disorders, including schizophrenia (see MCQ 2). TFTTT

Neurotic symptoms:

A. in twins, occur more commonly in the co-twin of affected individuals in monozygous compared with dizygous twins
B. are seldom precipitated by stressful life events
C. are more common in social adversity
D. are more common in those married women whose husbands show neurotic symptoms than in others
E. are mostly caused, according to research findings, by experiences in childhood

Important aetiological factors in the neuroses are those which place the individual under greater stress or make him or her more susceptible to the effects of stress. Such factors include social adversity, covering a range of specific problems like unemployment and inadequate or unsatisfactory social supports. Those patients who present to their general practitioners have an excess of life events in the three months before the onset of their symptoms. However, it is important to remember that not everyone who undergoes a stressful life event will develop neurotic symptoms or a neurotic illness—some individuals are more vulnerable than others.

Women whose husbands have neurotic symptoms are much more likely than other married women to develop neuroses themselves. The evidence suggests that the wife's symptoms are caused by living with a neurotic husband, because the longer the marriage, the greater the number of symptoms.

Twin studies have revealed a moderate degree of genetic predisposition. The concordance of symptoms is thus greater in monozygous twins than in dizygous twins (see MCQ 10).

Although a number of theories of the neuroses stress the importance of experiences in childhood, how precisely these relate to adult neurotic symptoms remains unclear. According to psychoanalytic theory, the predisposition to neurosis arises during childhood development—neurosis is the result of a failure in normal emotional development. Another view is that the neuroses represent particular forms of learned behaviour arising in childhood. None of the theories relating childhood experience to adult neurosis is without its pitfalls, and all have proved difficult to test through research. Although some childhood emotional problems persist into adulthood, when they often manifest themselves as neurotic symptoms, the vast majority of neurotic children do not become neurotic adults, and most adults with neuroses showed no evidence of neurotic symptoms when they were children (see MCQ 11). TFTTF

Neurotic disorders:

A. usually increase the risk of death by suicide or accidents
B. have a better prognosis in women than men
C. identified in the community often improve within six months of diagnosis
D. seen by psychiatrists have a similar prognosis to those seen by general practitioners
E. seen in general practice have a prognosis determined predominantly by the particular symptoms at presentation

Neurotic disorders have a variable prognosis. About half of cases identified in the community will recover within three months, while half of those seen in general practice will remain ill after one year. Only a minority of patients with neurosis seen by general practitioners are referred to psychiatrists. This group includes patients whose symptoms are more chronic and/or more severe and here, the outcome is less favourable. Of those patients with neurosis seen by psychiatrists, about half will remain symptomatic after four years.

Chronicity is the main prognostic indicator—longstanding symptoms at the time of presentation predict a poor outcome. Other unfavourable prognostic signs include severe symptoms at presentation, poor social supports and persistent social problems. A sound premorbid personality and the acute onset of symptoms in response to a temporary event suggest a more favourable outcome. Allowing for these other factors, prognosis is not significantly influenced by the sex of the patient. There are differences in prognosis between the specific neurotic syndromes, but for those neuroses seen in general practice (which comprise mainly undifferentiated neuroses—see MCQ 58) the precise symptoms at presentation do not significantly influence outcome.

Among neurotic patients, the risk of death from suicide or accidents increases by a factor of 1.5–2, although the presence of obsessional symptoms seems to protect against this. TFTFF

Anxiety neurosis:

A. has both psychological and physical symptoms
B. always involves a particular situation which generates excessive fear
C. may present with non-specific somatic symptoms
D. tends to cluster in families
E. should as a rule be treated with full doses of benzodiazepines for the duration of the illness

Anxiety states as defined by ICD9 are 'various combinations of physical and mental manifestations of anxiety, not attributable to real danger, and occurring either in attacks or as a persisting state. The anxiety is usually diffuse and may extend to panic. Other neurotic features may be present but do not dominate the clinical picture.'

Anxiety states constitute the most common specific neurotic disorder. Psychological symptoms include a persistent feeling of fearful anticipation, irritability, poor concentration and anxious ruminations. Physical symptoms result from sympathetic over-arousal and increased muscle tension and may include non-specific aches and pains as well as symptoms referable to the cardiovascular, genitourinary and gastrointestinal tracts. Weight loss and initial insomnia may occur. Overbreathing, with symptoms of hypocapnia, may present diagnostic problems (MCQ 116).

In some cases, the patient's anxiety is a response to a particular object or situation—**phobic anxiety** ★. In other cases, there is no specific phobic stimulus; this type of anxiety is sometimes termed **free-floating**. Free-floating anxiety often manifests as acute attacks of anxiety (**panic attacks**).

Anxiety neurosis tends to cluster in families. Twin studies have shown a greater genetic predisposition to anxiety neuroses than other neurotic syndromes. Other aetiological factors relevant to the neuroses as a whole also apply specifically to anxiety neurosis (see MCQ 59).

Attention to the details of the patient's complaints will often help to distinguish symptoms due to anxiety from those due to other causes. Thorough physical examination and appropriate investigations early in treatment will reassure both doctor and patient. Patients are commonly frightened and bewildered by the symptoms of anxiety—suffering the symptoms makes the anxiety worse, setting up a vicious circle. Helping the patient understand the symptoms, for example, by offering an explanation of the mechanisms and consequences of sympathetic over-arousal, is an important part of management and, in some cases, may be the only necessary intervention. Support, reassurance and attention to correctible social difficulties also form part of treatment. Treatment with anxiolytic drugs may be useful, but caution should be used in prescribing benzodiazepines because of their dependence potential and because of the apparent development of tolerance in some patients. As a rule, they should be used for only brief periods of time (one or two weeks) and usually as part of a treatment plan involving other components such as relaxation training. If more prolonged drug use is necessary, it may be preferable to use an antidepressant or even a antipsychotic drug in low dosage. There is evidence that panic disorders respond preferentially to treatment with antidepressants. Behavioural ★, cognitive ★ and relaxation techniques may be useful and there is anecdotal evidence for the efficacy in some patients of analytic (exploratory) psychotherapy ★.

The outcome of the anxiety neuroses is poor in those cases with a longer than six months' duration and a plethora of physical symptoms also adversely affects outcome. If the disorder is of short duration in an individual with a sound premorbid personality, recovery is likely. TFTTF

Which of the following statements are true regarding phobic disorders?

A. they lead to avoidance of the feared situation or object
B. the fear is out of proportion to the objective risk of the provoking situation
C. the patient loses insight into the excessive nature of his fear
D. animal phobias are not uncommon in childhood
E. the principle of treatment is exposure to the feared object or situation

Phobias are intense, irrational fears of a certain object or specific situations which would not normally have that effect. The patient realises that the fear is out of proportion to the situation (that is, retains insight into the nature of the symptom), but the fear is beyond voluntary control and leads to avoidance of the feared situation. The extent of this avoidance is a useful measure of the severity of the phobia. For example, some people will completely avoid travelling on buses, while for others, it is possible to travel by bus provided that the bus is not too crowded and that they can find a seat near the door or emergency exit.

Phobias can be classified into **simple** (or **specific** phobias, in which the fear is focused on a specific object, **social phobia** ★, in which there is an irrational fear of social situations, and **agoraphobia** ★, in which there is an abnormal fear of crowded public places. Of these, agoraphobia is the most common. Agoraphobia and social phobia tend to be more complex than the specific phobias and consequently more difficult to treat.

Specific phobias may be further subdivided into **animal phobias** (in which the feared object is an animal, commonly spider, dog, bird or moth) and **miscellaneous specific phobias** such as fear of enclosed spaces (**claustrophobia**), fear of death (**necrophobia**) or fear of heights (**acrophobia**). Animal phobias are not uncommon during childhood but tend to be relatively mild and transient.

The principle of treatment of the phobias is **exposure** to the feared object or situation. This can be carried out gradually (**systematic desensitisation** ★, in which the patient is taken up a hierarchy of feared situations—a 'little-by-little' approach (see MCQ 133). Alternatively, in **flooding (implosion** ★), the patient is 'thrown in at the deep end' and exposed to a situation high up on his hierarchy from the beginning. Exposure is best carried in real life (in vivo) but if this is impossible or impracticable (e.g. in fear of flying), it can be done in imagination. Relaxation techniques and encouragement may help the patient through the difficult phases of treatment (although some experts consider that relaxation makes no significant contribution to behaviour therapy programmes) but tranquillisers are best avoided since there is some evidence that they impede behavioural change. Phobias may occur in the setting of a depressive illness, in which case this should be treated before behavioural treatment is started. TTFTT

Agoraphobia:

A. is an abnormally intense dread of open spaces
B. is commoner in females than males
C. may severely restrict social activity
D. is frequently accompanied by depression
E. is usually easily treated by desensitisation

'Agora' usually means marketplace—agoraphobia is phobia of busy public places. The characteristic symptoms are panic attacks or persistent anxiety occurring in relation to crowded streets, shops and public transport, such that the patient progressively avoids such situations. Such situations have in common the fact that the person has nowhere to hide or escape, or find reassurance, in the event of a panic attack. When mild, the patient may still be able to venture out alone but avoid places like supermarkets. As the symptoms become more severe, going outdoors may only be possible in the company of a relative or friend, and in severe cases the person becomes completely housebound, feeling unable to go out at all. Agoraphobia is commoner in women than men, and is often accompanied by depressive symptoms. Obsessional symptoms and depersonalisation may also occur.

The aetiology of agoraphobia is unknown, although the condition is commonly accompanied by marital or sexual problems. There is little evidence of a genetic predisposition. Psychoanalytic theories suggest a displacement or projection of fears or anxieties from internal (often sexual) conflicts to the external world.

The condition usually begins in the third or fourth decade and may run a chronic course. Behavioural treatments concentrating on self-exposure or therapist-assisted exposure are the treatments of choice and may prove highly effective, with low relapse rates in some cases. In other cases, treatment is more difficult (for example, getting the patient's or the spouse's cooperation with treatment might prove difficult) and here the disorder may prove intractable, becoming a way of life. Tricyclic antidepressants and monoamine oxidase inhibitors may reduce both depressive and agoraphobic symptoms, but there is a high relapse rate on drug withdrawal. FTTTF

Social phobia:

A. is a sub-type of agoraphobia
B. is equally common in men and women
C. is a severe form of social inadequacy
D. usually responds favourably to social skills training
E. may be accompanied by excessive intake of alcohol

Social phobia is a fear of being scrutinised by other people. The social phobic believes that others are carefully watching him or her and picking up all his or her inadequacies. In addition to the common features of anxiety, people with social phobia often feel that they blush or perspire excessively, or that they have a tremor, which others can easily recognise. The distinction between agoraphobia and social phobia rests with the phobic stimulus—particular types of place in the former, people in the latter. An agoraphobic can usually identify settings in which she is comfortable in the presence of others (notably at home) while the social phobic may feel this way with only a handful of close friends, regardless of the setting. Careful attention to the patient's own description of his problems helps to distinguish these two types of phobia. For example, a social phobic might even have difficulty talking on the telephone, although this is not a feature of agoraphobia. However, some of the behaviours involved in the two phobias might overlap. For example, like agoraphobics, social phobics might be unable to leave the house alone but in the latter case, having someone else there is intended as a safeguard against having to talk to someone one might meet, rather than any other fear.

Despite the (irrational) fear that others are watching one's every move, social phobics do not necessarily lack social skills and may in the past have shown no evidence of social inadequacy.

Social phobia is equally common in both sexes and usually starts between the ages of 17 and 30. It is not uncommon for people with social phobia to use alcohol in attempting to overcome their fears, and the condition is sometimes accompanied by excessive use of alcohol. Depression is another possible accompaniment of social phobia.

Treatment is along behavioural lines, by graded exposure to a series of increasingly difficult social situations. Cognitive techniques ★ may also prove very helpful. Where the patient is married, it is often appropriate and important to involve the spouse in the therapy. Other accompanying problems, such as alcoholism or depression, require assessment and management in their own right. FTFFT

MCQ 65

Obsessive-compulsive disorder (neurosis):

A. is a common disorder
B. is more common in females than males
C. always involves compulsive rituals
D. often undergoes exacerbations and remissions
E. often responds poorly to treatment

The essential feature of obsessive-compulsive disorder is the occurrence of obsessions ★, which occur with sufficient frequency significantly to interfere with normal functioning and, when extreme, may be incapacitating.

Obsessional symptoms may take the form of simple thoughts or fears or more complex ruminations, in which the person might endlessly and pointlessly review even the simplest everyday event. In **obsessional doubting**, there is recurrent questioning of acts that have already been, or are about to be, carried out. Such activity can lead to **obsessional slowness** with everyday tasks taking a long time to complete.

Obsessional acts are called compulsions ★, which may be organised into complicated and disabling rituals. Not all obsessional disorders involve compulsions. The need to perform compulsive rituals may be another reason for slowness in a patient with this disorder. For example, a patient may need to wash his face in a particular way, starting precisely at the same point each time, always moving the flannel clockwise a certain number of times, making sure that the soap is placed in precisely the right position, and so on. If the ritual is interrupted, or if it does not follow precisely the correct sequence (like the soap slipping, in the above example), the patient may feel compelled to begin the whole ritual again. Such rituals can occupy many hours of each day.

Although obsessional symptoms are not uncommon in other psychiatric disorders, 'pure' obsessive-compulsive disorder is rare. One-year prevalence rates vary between 0.1 and 2.0 per 1000. The disorder occurs equally frequently in both sexes and the peak age of onset is in the third decade. Rarely, obsessional symptoms may accompany organic brain syndromes such as space-occupying lesions, which may need to be excluded.

The course is characterised by remissions and exacerbations, and treatment is usually difficult, especially when the patient has no compulsions. The latter may be amenable to behavioural techniques such as stopping the patient carrying out the ritual (**response prevention**). Where depression is present, this requires treatment in its own right. It is sometimes possible to treat obsessional thoughts by distraction or thought stopping (for example, by getting the patient to wear a thick elastic band on the wrist and pulling the band hard then releasing it whenever the ruminations start). FFFTT

The term 'hysteria' or 'hysterical' may be correctly used to denote:

A. symptoms and signs of disease produced unconsciously in the absence of organic pathology
B. symptoms and signs of disease, consciously produced in order to achieve some gain
C. a syndrome, usually occurring in females, with persistent physical symptoms affecting a variety of organ systems
D. an epidemic of physical symptoms, with no apparent organic cause, occurring in members of an institution
E. a personality type characterised by theatricality, shallow relationships, a self-centred approach to life and a craving for excitement

Hysteria involves alteration in bodily function or in level of consciousness which is not due to an underlying physical cause. The signs and symptoms are produced unconsciously. In practice, it may be difficult to distinguish hysteria from **malingering ★**, also characterised by somatic symptoms and signs in the absence of any underlying physical cause, but where the signs are produced consciously, and the patient fully aware of what he is doing. It is customary to subdivide hysteria into **hysterical conversion ★** and **hysterical dissociation ★**. The former involves disturbances of motor or sensory function (for example, paralysis, anaesthesiae), the latter disturbances of consciousness (notably hysterical amnesia).

Briquet's syndrome is the name applied to a form of hysteria involving predominantly female patients who, before the age of 30, develop multiple physical symptoms involving several organ systems with no evidence of any underlying physical cause(s). The condition persists and frequently results in repeated medical and surgical interventions.

Epidemic hysteria is a curious and uncommon condition occurring usually in institutions, like schools. It usually begins with a susceptible individual developing (hysterical) signs or symptoms, which rapidly spread to other members of the institution. The condition may disappear when members of the affected institution are separated.

The **hysterical (histrionic) personality disorder** is characterised by overdramatisation, attention-seeking behaviour, shallow relationships and emotional lability with extreme egocentricity. The sufferers may appear attractive or seductive but have little enjoyment in life, leading to depression and deliberate self-harm. In common with other personality disorders ★, this is a not a very reliable diagnosis, and can sometimes be seen as a perjorative label. For these reasons, it is probably best avoided. TFTTT

In hysterical conversion:

A. signs and symptoms of apparent neurological disease are often present
B. there is never underlying physical disease
C. some patients will develop serious medical or neurological disorders
D. it is presumed that real or imagined gain accrues from the symptoms
E. there may be relative lack of concern considering the often serious handicap caused by the symptoms

In hysterical conversion (conversion disorder), signs and symptoms of physical disorder are present. These are not due to underlying organic pathology, but are presumed to be due to an unconscious psychological conflict. The commonest symptoms mimic neurological disorders, such as paralysis or paresis, aphonia, seizures, blindness or sensory disturbances. Characteristically, the symptoms do not follow the pattern expected from physiological or anatomical considerations. An example of this would be a 'glove and stocking' sensory deficit. However, diagnosis is sometimes complicated by the presence of a (coincident) physical disorder. Although the hysterical signs are presumed to have no organic basis, it is important not to assume from this that all the patient's complaints are due to hysteria. Thorough physical examination is always necessary and further investigations may be appropriate. Even when no organic pathology is detected, the diagnosis of hysteria cannot be held with complete certainty. A small minority of patients diagnosed as having hysteria go on during long-term follow-up to manifest physical illness, presumed to have been the cause of the original symptoms but not initially detectable.

Hysterical conversion is rare in modern psychiatric practice but tends to present to neurologists and sometimes to other physicians. The condition often arises in the setting of depression or severe stress. Psychoanalytic theories emphasise the presumed unconscious mechanisms involving primary and sometimes also secondary gain. The patient is considered to have a painful internal conflict, which the hysterical symptoms serve to suppress—this is **primary gain**. For example, a young woman who feels torn between staying with her boyfriend and ending the relationship, and who then develops hysterical paralysis of both legs, no longer needs to address her conflict about running away. Coming into hospital, she gets attention and sympathy from family and friends—this is **secondary gain**. Secondary gain is not directly linked to the hysterical symptoms. Friends, relatives and others are often aware of secondary gains but tend to be oblivious to primary gain. Although primary and secondary gain are most commonly linked with hysteria, they are in fact features of all the neuroses.

The patient often appears relatively unconcerned about the symptoms, even when they give rise to serious handicaps. This is termed **la belle indifférence**.

In principle, treatment involves attempting to understand and remove the gain while minimising the sick role. Early intervention is advisable, because if the symptoms become chronic they may prove intractable and can give rise to secondary complications. For example, someone with hysterical paralysis of a leg might develop flexion contractures. On acute presentation, it is worth considering a trial of abreaction, in which a slow intravenous infusion of diazepam or amylobarbitone is given to disinhibit the patient without excessive sedation. Under these conditions, encouraging the patient to 'relive' the experience that is presumed to have given rise to the symptoms may lead to the symptoms improving or even disappearing completely. However, how abreaction works (and indeed whether it works at all) remains controversial—in some cases, the use of suggestion alone is successful (for example, 'after this injection, you ought to be able to get just a little movement in one of your toes and we can go on from there'). TFTTT

In dissociative disorders (hysterical dissociation):

A. amnesia is usually total
B. the disorder can sometimes be traced to abnormalities in the reticular activating system
C. perplexity and disorientation are uncommon
D. depersonalisation and derealisation may occur
E. the phenomenon of multiple personality has been described

In **hysterical (psychogenic) amnesia** there is a sudden loss of memory, not due to any organic cause. The amnesia may be circumscribed and affects recall for hours to days around some profoundly disturbing event. It may be selective for certain events during a period of time. Alternatively, it may be total and global, so that the patient is unable to recall anything at all about himself. Psychogenic amnesia should also be suspected when the patient shows profound amnesia for all past events but no significant deficit in forming new memories. As in other forms of amnesia, perplexity and disorientation may occur.

Fugue states are rare phenomena characterised by wandering behaviour together with amnesia. During a psychogenic fugue, the individual may even take on a new identity. Evidence of gain is commonly apparent. Note that hysteria is not the only cause of fugue states. These may occur in epilepsy and secondary to alcoholism.

Multiple personality is a rare condition in which an individual possesses two or more distinct personalities, although only one is predominant at any given time. Each personality is an apparently fully integrated 'unit' which functions in a particular role. Transition from one personality to another may occur suddenly in response to stress and each personality may be unaware of the existence of the others. However, the nature of this phenomenon has not been adequately elucidated and some authorities remain sceptical about its existence.

A more common dissociative disorder is **depersonalisation**. This is a sense that one is 'unreal'. The body (or parts of it) are experienced as unreal, remote or altered in quality in some other way. This phenomenon is not uncommon in the general population, especially associated with stress (such as walking into an examination hall) but is considered pathological if it occurs with sufficient severity or frequency to interfere with normal functioning. Depersonalisation also occurs in anxiety and depression, and may sometimes be seen in psychotic disorders. Depersonalisation may be accompanied by **derealisation**, the sense that one's surroundings are not real. People who experience this sometimes talk of their surrounding looking as if they were 'cardboard cutouts' of real objects or people, or that everything looks like a stage set. FFFTT

Hypochondriasis:

A. is an abnormal preoccupation with bodily health or disease
B. should not be diagnosed if organic disease is present
C. may occur as part of a depressive disorder
D. responds to reassurance
E. is a form of obsessional neurosis, since it involves repetitive intrusive thoughts about health or disease which interfere with normal functioning

Hypochondriasis, like hysteria, is a difficult term to define accurately. It involves a morbid preoccupation with health (or disease) out of proportion to existing justification, usually accompanied by persistent attempts to seek reassurance. The main problem with this definition lies with the difficulty in deciding at what point a person's preoccupation with some aspect of bodily functioning becomes disproportionate and therefore pathological. This is often difficult to determine, except in the most extreme cases. 'Hypochondriasis' has, as a result, come to assume a pejorative meaning, as a term applied by some doctors, to a particular kind of 'difficult' patient. Some authorities prefer to use the term **abnormal illness behaviour** to emphasise the behavioural aspects of the disorder.

Hypochondriasis involves repetitive and intrusive thoughts (about health and/or disease), and to this extent, it resembles obsessive-compulsive disorder. However, the fundamental distinction between these is that obsessions are recognised by the sufferer as senseless, while in hypochondriasis, the ruminations about disease are regarded as true and appropriate. Pain is the most common symptom, and gastrointestinal, cardiovascular and respiratory symptoms are also frequent. Given the opportunity, hypochondriacal patients often talk at length about the symptoms they suffer, their physiological functions and so on (the 'organ recital'). Hypochondriasis may coexist with organic illness, further complicating diagnosis and management.

Most commonly, hypochondriasis occurs in the setting of another disorder, like depression, anxiety or schizophrenia (secondary hypochondriasis). Whether primary hypochondriasis exists at all remains the subject of debate. Because of the difficulty in making this diagnosis accurately, the prevalence of hypochondriasis is uncertain. However, estimates of the proportion of patients consulting doctors with what might be hypochondriacal complaints vary from 30% to 80%.

The aetiology of hypochondriasis is complex and poorly understood. Past experience of (organic) illness, either oneself or in a close relative, predisposes to hypochondriasis. In this respect, it is interesting to note that hypochondriasis may be a feature of bereavement ★, when it sometimes presents with symptoms similar to those suffered by the person who died. Psychodynamic theories have attempted to account for the condition in terms of either an alternative channel through which to deflect basic drives (sexual, aggressive, and so on) or as a defence mechanism against guilt or low self-esteem.

Management can be difficult. Treatment of another underlying or concomitant psychiatric disorder is important. By definition, hypochondriasis shows no persistent response to reassurance, although this may offer temporary respite. A prerequisite for successful treatment is to 'engage' the patient, which involves taking his symptoms seriously and particularly trying to understand the symptoms and preoccupations from the patient's point of view. Unless this is achieved, the patient will move on to another doctor to seek a satisfactory outcome. Not uncommonly, hypochondriacal patients see numerous doctors simultaneously and build up very thick medical casenotes. Careful and detailed explanation of the nature of the symptoms sometimes helps (note that this is not the same as reassuring the patient that there is nothing seriously wrong). Anxiety is frequently present and may exacerbate the somatic symptoms; here, anxiety management using relaxation and other methods may prove valuable. A cognitive approach may also be very helpful, for example in identifying the patient's beliefs about his health and then examining the available evidence for and against those beliefs. TFTFF

Personality Disorders

MCQ 70

Personality disorders:

A. usually pervade every aspect of the individual's functioning within society
B. are usually diagnosed with greater emphasis on details gethered from the person's observed behaviour than on past history
C. most commonly become manifest in the third decade
D. include personalities which are conspicuously different from 'normal' but do not have adverse effects either on the individual or on society
E. have a well-established genetic predisposition

Personality disorders are maladaptive abnormalities of personality which cause either the patient or others to suffer and have an adverse effect on the individual and/or society. An important characteristic of all personality disorders is that the abnormality should have been present since an early age (childhood or early adolescence) and remains evident throughout adult life. In addition, the abnormality is persistent, with an often conspicuous failure to learn from experience. The abnormalities may affect the whole personality, or only discrete parts of it. An example of the latter might be someone who is very successful professionally but is quite incapable of sustaining close personal relationships. Even when severe, such abnormalities do not necessarily pervade the whole personality and the individuals concerned may in some respects function very well within society.

By no means all abnormal personalities come into the category of personality disorders. Someone who is very eccentric, for example, may be recognised as having a personality which differs widely from the norm, but may not, because of this personality, cause distress or suffering to himself or to anyone else. Indeed, some eccentrics have personalities which could not be described even as maladaptive. Conversely, not everyone who causes suffering to himself or others warrants this diagnosis. Someone who has committed a violent crime may show no evidence of past abnormal personality and here, the diagnosis of personality disorder is inappropriate.

Given the features of personality disorders described above, it is not surprising that more emphasis is placed in diagnosis on the individual's past history than on his present behaviour or overall mental state. Even then, the diagnosis poses considerable problems, notably due to the obvious difficulties in defining the 'normal' personality and its limits. For this reason, the diagnosis of personality disorder is often unreliable, and care must be taken in using it. Both ICD9 ★ and DSM-IIIR ★ subdivide personality disorders into different types, but these subtypes are even less reliable to use in practice, and there is often considerable overlap between one subtype and others. However, one specific sub-type is particularly important—the antisocial (psychopathic) personality disorder ★.

Aetiology is unclear. There is some evidence from twin studies for a genetic component in the inheritance of personality attributes, but a genetic basis for personality disorders remains to be firmly established. Psychoanalytic theories suggest that personality may become disordered if the individual fails to pass through the normal stages of emotional development in early childhood. This may offer a conceptual framework which fits some individual cases, but is very difficult to test more widely. Disturbances in parent-child relationships have been implicated in the aetiology of antisocial personality disorder and may also influence the development of other types of disordered personality.

By definition, personality disorders are resistant to change, and management is thus difficult. The main principles in management are not to be overly ambitious in one's therapeutic aims and to take care and effort in negotiating appropriate limits with the individual who presents—how often the appointments will be, how long each will last, what you will expect to do during the appointments, and so on. Some people with personality disorders may become dependent on a doctor (or anyone else who shows interest and concern)—the likelihood and effects of this may be minimised by making a firm contract and sticking to it. Sometimes, it is appropriate to offer no more than regular support. In other instances, focused therapy on specific problems might be helpful.

Long-term exploratory psychotherapy may be appropriate for selected younger individuals. In general, drugs have very little part to play in management. However, people with disordered personalities may at some time become clinically depressed or manifest other psychiatric disorders, and these should be treated in the usual way.

Whether personality disorder should be seen as an 'illness' or 'psychiatric disorder' is also controversial. Many psychiatrists argue that the personality disorders are not psychiatric illnesses and, because psychiatry has little expertise to offer affected individuals, such people are not followed up in their clinics. However, some understanding of personality disorder is important for general practitioners and other doctors, to whom people with personality disorders may present. FFFFF

Antisocial (psychopathic/sociopathic) personality disorder:

A. is easily treatable in specialised units
B. is characterised by an apparent lack of a sense of guilt or conscience
C. results in repeated antisocial or criminal behaviour
D. is associated with a higher than expected incidence of non-specific EEG abnormalities
E. tends to cluster in families

This condition is defined in ICD9 as 'a personality disorder characterised by disregard for social obligations, lack of feeling for others, and impetuous violence or callous unconcern. There is a gross disparity between behaviour and the prevailing social norms. Behaviour is not readily modifiable by experience, including punishment. People with this personality are often affectively cold and may be abnormally aggressive or irresponsible. Their tolerance to frustration is low; they blame others or offer plausible rationalisations for the behaviour which brings them into conflict with society.'

Various theories have been proposed to explain why some people habitually behave in antisocial or impulsive ways but none of the available theories is satisfactory. The condition tends to cluster in families characterised by social disturbance, disruption and often alcohol abuse in other members of the family. Prospective studies have revealed that repeated delinquent behaviour in children is a powerful predictor of antisocial behaviour in adulthood. In about 40% of antisocial children the condition will persist into adulthood. One third to one half of individuals with this diagnosis show non-specific EEG abnormalities such as slow waves (in the temporal leads or more generally distributed) or fast sharp wave activity over the temporal lobes. These findings resemble EEG patterns occurring normally in children and this has led to the concept of 'cortical immaturity' in people with this diagnosis. Sociopathic behaviour does appear to lessen with age in some instances.

As with personality disorders in general, a major problem in discussing this disorder is the lack of reliable diagnostic criteria and research is bedevilled by each author's particular conceptualisation of the syndrome. Treatment is difficult, even in specialist units. FTTTT

The Munchausen syndrome:

A. is also called the hospital addiction syndrome
B. is a form of conversion hysteria
C. is also known as malingering
D. characteristically involves patients moving from hospital to hospital simulating serious illness
E. commonly responds well to psychotherapy

The 'hospital addiction syndrome' (Munchausen syndrome), described by Asher in 1951, owes its name to Baron von Münchhausen, a fictitious character famous for his fantastic stories of adventure.

The characteristic feature of people with the Munchausen syndrome is their inexplicable need to move from one hospital to the next, fabricating dramatic signs and symptoms of physical illness, only to disappear when confronted by their deceit. Any combination of symptoms may be simulated, but presentations resembling myocardial infarction, renal colic or an acute abdomen are probably the most common. Patients sometimes go to extreme lengths to convince professionals of their illness, for example adding blood to urine samples to simulate haematuria, or swallowing then regurgitating blood to simulate haematemesis. Other bizarre behaviour includes the swallowing of spoons to simulate intestinal obstruction or the surreptitious opening of sugical scars. Such behaviour often indicates considerable medical knowledge, and some patients have a medical or paramedical background. Others are able to piece together salient signs and symptoms during repeated admissions to different hospitals, often using different names.

The condition appears to be a chronic maladaptive pattern of behaviour and some patients have had literally hundreds of admissions and several surgical procedures. The cause of this extraordinary behaviour is obscure. The condition is probably best thought of as a type of abnormal illness behaviour produced consciously for the purpose of gain, although the benefits of such behaviour to the patient are often difficult to understand. Possibly, the dramatic deceiving of hospital personnel, and medical attention, act as reinforcers.

In the Munchausen syndrome, the symptoms and signs are produced consciously and deliberately. This is the fundamental difference between this disorder and hysteria, in which the symptoms and signs are presumed to be unconscious ★. In practice, this distinction may be difficult to make. In **malingering** ★ the patient again presents with signs and symptoms of illness which are consciously produced. However, here there is usually a particular purpose behind the feigned illness, commonly to gain compensation or to avoid an unpleasant situation (as, for example, in the case of a man on remand in prison awaiting trial). Patients who are malingering are not expected to go on to manifest the Munchausen syndrome.

Variants of the syndrome include **Munchausen by proxy**, in which someone deliberately simulates illness in another person, for example another member of the family. Most commonly, a mother will present with an 'ill' child. This may in some cases constitute child abuse ★. 'Psychiatric Munchausen' syndrome is the simulation of psychiatric disorder—such patients usually claim to have auditory hallucinations.

Patients with this syndrome commonly discharge themselves against medical advice. This often follows arguments with staff, particularly after the patient has been confronted with his deceit. It is thus difficult to form a therapeutic relationship. Management is thus focused on early detection. Past history as given by the patient is commonly vague or may even be contradictory. It is also difficult to sustain consistently abnormal symptoms and signs, and such inconsistency may be revealed by careful observation. TFFTF

Substance Abuse and Dependence

MCQ 73

Which of the following statements about excessive alcohol consumption are true?

A. an essential feature of alcoholism is **physical** dependence on alcohol
B. a man who every day consumes more than the equivalent of 50 g of absolute alcohol is very likely to be an alcoholic or to become one
C. someone may be defined as alcoholic who continues to drink in spite of incurring physical or psychological damage as a result of alcohol
D. having to take a drink first thing in the morning is an indication of alcohol dependence
E. a man who drinks beer is less likely to become an alcoholic than one who drinks spirits

Consumption of alcohol is best described in terms of '**standard units**', one of which is equivalent to approximately 10 g of absolute alcohol. One half-pint of bitter, a single tot of spirits, one glass of sherry and a glass of wine are each approximately equivalent to one standard unit. The Royal College of Psychiatrists has suggested that reasonable upper limits of alcohol consumption are the equivalent of 60 g of absolute alcohol daily for men and 30 g daily for women. However, the definition of what constitutes 'excessive' consumpton of alcohol varies, as does the level of drinking which may be considered 'safe'. This is one reason why it is unsatisfactory to define alcoholism purely in terms of the amount of alcohol consumed. There are numerous available definitions of alcoholism. Two features common to most of these definitions of alcoholism are that drinking is excessive *and* that drinking results in serious or persistent disabilities or problems for the drinker and/or other people. There is no evidence that one type of alcoholic drink is more likely than another to lead to alcoholism.

A concept related to alcoholism is that of **alcohol dependence**. Features of the alcohol dependence syndrome include a compulsion to drink, the predominance of drinking over other activities, and altered tolerance to alcohol. Also important are repeated withdrawal symptoms, which involve shakiness, sweating, nausea, irritability and dysphoria and may progress to delirium tremens ★. Such withdrawal symptoms may be relieved or avoided by further drinking. Thus someone who suffers from the alcohol dependence syndrome may need to have alcohol at his bedside to drink immediately on awakening. Most people drink in response to certain social cues, such as going to the pub with friends or having wine with a meal. A further feature of the alcohol dependence syndrome is the development of a stereotyped pattern of drinking based not on such social cues but only on the need to relieve or avoid withdrawal symptoms. This is termed 'narrowing of the drinking repertoire'. Those who are severely dependent on alcohol are also likely, after a period of abstinence, to relapse into their old pattern of drinking when they take one or two drinks.

Alcoholism and alcohol dependence are not synonymous. While all those who manifest the alcohol dependence syndrome are alcoholics, the converse is not true. FFTTF

The prevalence of alcoholism:

A. is high in countries where per capita consumption of alcohol is high
B. is lowest in socioeconomic class I
C. in children whose parent(s) are alcoholic and who have been adopted away from their parents in early life is no greater than in adopted children without alcoholic parents
D. is low among doctors
E. is greatest in individuals with neurasthenic personalities

Estimates of the prevalence of alcoholism depend on how alcoholism is defined (see MCQ 73) and on the method of ascertaining cases. Epidemiological surveys suggest a prevalence rate among English adults of approximately 6 per 1000 for males and 1.5 per 1000 for females. However, estimates of alcoholism based on self-report measures can be very unreliable. To overcome this problem, a number of methods have been used to assess the prevalence of alcoholism indirectly. For example, a significant positive correlation has been found between mortality from liver cirrhosis and the per capita consumption of alcohol. This relationship holds not only at different times within one country but also between countries—those countries with greater per capita consumption of alcohol also have higher mortality rates from cirrhosis. Hospital admission rates for alcoholism provide another indirect indicator of prevalence, although these are influenced by hospital admission policies. In Scotland, admission rates for alcoholism are seven times greater for males and five times greater for females than they are in England and Wales.

The peak age group of alcoholics is from the early 40's to mid-50's. The ratio of men to women affected is 2.5:1, but the prevalence of alcoholism is increasing more rapidly in women than in men. Lowest prevalence is found in the middle class. The divorced and separated of both sexes together with unmarried women face a higher risk. Certain occupational groups such as company directors, doctors, journalists, commercial travellers and those in the liquor trade are particularly prone. These occupations share several characteristics, including relative absence of regular workplace, lack or absence of supervision, ready availability of alcohol and subcultural encouragement of drinking. Ethnic influence is apparent in the high rates found in American Blacks and the Irish and low rates in Jews. Alcoholism is also being increasingly recognised as a growing problem among the elderly. Among those whose excessive drinking begins in later life, factors contributing to the onset of alcoholism include the changes in role and personal status associated with retirement, bereavement and increasing social isolation.

These patterns of prevalence indicate the relevance of sociocultural factors in the aetiology of alcoholism. Biological and psychological factors are also important. Children fostered or adopted away when very young from alcoholic parents have a four times greater risk of developing alcoholism than adopted children whose biological parents were not alcoholic, suggesting that genetic factors may also contribute. Frank psychiatric illness is common among alcoholics and may contribute in some cases to the development of alcoholism. In other cases, the psychiatric disturbance may be an effect of the alcoholism rather than a cause. No specific personality type has been associated consistently with the development of alcoholism but there is some evidence to suggest that aggressive and antisocial traits in childhood may be associated with later alcoholism. TFFFF

Which of the following have recognised associations with alcoholism?

A. auditory hallucinations in clear consciousness, with no other features of psychosis
B. deliberate self-harm
C. morbid jealousy
D. microcytosis without anaemia
E. exhibitionism

It is convenient to classify the problems and disabilities associated with alcoholism into three groups—physical, psychological and social.

Physical problems associated with alcoholism include cirrhosis, peptic ulceration and damage to the brain and nervous tissue (see MCQ 76). Pregnant women who are alcoholics are likely to have children who show the foetal alcohol syndrome, with decreased birthweight, small head circumference, mental retardation and a numerous other congenital defects. Anaemia and vitamin deficiencies may be found. Withdrawal from alcohol may result in delirium tremens ★. Laboratory tests which may be useful in the detection of alcoholism before it becomes fully manifest include liver function tests (particularly gamma-glutamyl transpeptidase levels) and full blood count, which may reveal a macrocytic picture even in the absence of anaemia (see MCQ 77).

Alcoholism is associated with an increased prevalence of functional psychiatric disorders, although it is often difficult to decide whether these are the cause or the result of the alcoholism. Irritability and dysphoria are common and may be mistaken for a depressive illness. Alcohol is commonly consumed before acts of deliberate self-harm and approximately 10–15% of completed suicides have a previous history of alcoholism. A variety of sexual problems can occur, including impotence, and acts of exhibitionism or indecency due in some cases to the disinhibitant effects of alcohol. Alcohol is a common concomitant of marital violence, with approximately 50% of battered wives reporting their husbands as heavy drinkers. **Morbid jealousy** ★ is another association of alcoholism, in which the patient has a delusional belief that his spouse or partner is unfaithful to him. This is an important diagnosis to make because of the potential danger to the partner of the patient acting on his feelings of jealousy. **Alcoholic hallucinosis** is a rare complication in which the patient has auditory hallucinations in clear consciousness—this commonly resolves after a few days' abstinence. Amnesic episodes and dementia (see MCQ 76) may also occur.

Alcoholism has numerous social consequences. Alcoholics lose more than twice as many days off work as the general working population. Alcoholics have three times as many accidents at home and at work as other people, and one in three drivers involved in road traffic accidents in Britain has a blood alcohol level in excess of the legal limit. 40% of prison inmates may be classified as excessive drinkers and alcoholism is associated with a wide variety of crimes, from petty theft to crimes of violence. TTTFT

MCQ 76

Neuropsychiatric complications of alcoholism include:

A. Wernicke's encephalopathy
B. Korsakoff's psychosis
C. dementia
D. amnesic episodes
E. epilepsy

Acute alcohol intoxication may occasionally lead to periods of dense amnesia ('**alcoholic blackouts**') during which the affected individual may carry out quite elaborate activities, but have no recollection of them later on. Such episodes may last several hours, and are thought to be related to rapid rise in blood alcohol concentration. Other effects of intoxication include stupor, coma and epilepsy. The latter however more commonly arises as a complication of withdrawal or as a consequence of brain damage produced by severe and prolonged alcohol consumption.

Direct toxic effects of alcohol may lead to cerebellar degeneration, polyneuropathy and diffuse cortical cell loss giving rise to dementia. However, this '**alcoholic dementia**' may be distinguished from other forms of dementia such as Alzheimer's disease in that progression is not inevitable and cognition may even improve with abstinence from alcohol. In addition to the direct toxic effects of alcohol on the brain, neuropsychiatric complications of alcoholism may arise as a result of associated nutritional dificiencies or as a result of withdrawal after established physical dependence.

Deficiency of thiamine (Vitamin B1) leads to Wernicke's encephalopathy ★. This usually resolves with thiamine replacement but may lead in a proportion of cases, especially if treatment is inadequate, to Korsakoff's psychosis ★.

Withdrawal phenomena may range in severity from isolated symptoms such as headache, tinnitus, hyperacusis and tremulousness to established delirium tremens ★. If left untreated, delirium tremens carries a high mortality. TTTTT

Regarding the detection and management of alcoholism:

A. elevated serum levels of gamma-glutamyl transpeptidase are a unreliable indicator of alcoholism
B. patients admitted to a medical ward with alcohol-related problems are unlikely to reduce their drinking without outpatient follow-up and supervision
C. the only reliable aim of treatment of alcoholism is complete absention from alcohol
D. patients who drink excessively who present to their general practitioner show alcohol-related problems or disabilities in the majority of cases
E. the patient's own estimate of his alcohol consumption is usually a reliable indicator of the extent of alcohol-related problems

20% or more of male medical inpatients have a history of excessive drinking or frank alcoholism. However, there is evidence that many of these patients with drink problems go undetected, both in hospital and when they present to general practitioners. Among hospital admissions, alcoholics often show evidence of alcohol-related diagnoses, like liver damage, peptic ulceration, oesophagitis, pancreatitis and epileptic fits. However, only the minority of patients who drink excessively and who present to their general practitioners show these and other alcohol-related problems such as absenteeism from work, an excess of accidents, and so on.

The detection of alcoholism depends on maintaining a high index of suspicion when taking histories from patients and on asking appropriate questions. Although research studies have shown that self-reported estimates of alcohol consumption can be reliable, patients tend to report that they drink less than they actually do. This is particularly likely among whose who drink excessively. Getting the patient to complete a 'drink diary'—a day-by-day account of his alcohol consumption over the recent past—is more accurate. In addition, a number of screening questions are helpful. Four questions commonly used, which make up the 'CAGE' questionnaire, are: 'Have you ever felt you should **C**ut down on your drinking?'; 'Have people **A**nnoyed you by criticising your drinking?'; 'Have you ever felt bad or **G**uilty about your drinking?'; 'Have you ever had a drink first thing in the morning (an **E**ye opener)?' Two or more positive answers to these questions suggest a diagnosis of alcoholism. Laboratory investigations may provide further evidence of alcoholism but are no substitute for an adequate history and clinical examination. The blood film commonly shows a raised mean corpuscular volume (MCV) and serum gamma-glutamyl transpeptidase (gamma-GT) levels may be elevated. However, gamma-GT levels rise in response to acute drinking binges even in the absence of chronic excessive alcohol intake.

Managment must be tailored to the particular problems, needs and resources of each individual patient. Excessive consumption of alcohol is usually only one of the problems the patient faces, and attempting to deal with the drinking in isolation often leads to treatment failure. There is no evidence that all alcoholics necessarily require specialist treatment. A recent study of medical inpatients with alcoholism showed that counselling the patients about the effects of alcohol during their admissions showed favourable effects on drinking one year later, without any specific follow-up. In treating alcoholics in general practice, it is worth establishing an individual treatment plan, comprising a series of short-term goals, negotiated by doctor and patient, aimed at reducing the amount of alcohol consumed, and finding alternative strategies to tackle the patient's other problems.

Withdrawal symptoms can be treated with diazepam or chlormethiazole given in a short course of descending dosage. It is important that such treatment is adequately supervised, because these drugs may be substituted for alcohol if they are taken for too long a time. Vitamins are often worth giving. Other drugs have only a minor role to play in management. A small minority of patients benefit from disulfiram or citrated calcium carbimide, as deterrents to impulsive drinking. These drugs interact with alcohol to give a range of unpleasant physical effects but are suitable only for use by those who are well motivated. A drinking binge on top of treatment with one of these drugs may even result in death. Patients who are more seriously dependent on alcohol are usually referred for specialist treatment, with inpatient detoxification if necessary. Many patients also benefit from contact with voluntary agencies such as Alcoholics Anonymous.

It used to be held that the only appropriate goal in the treatment of alcoholism was complete abstinence. For some patients (particularly those who are seriously dependent on alcohol, over 40 years old and with few social supports) this may be the only reliable way of dealing with their alcoholism. However, others are able to return to controlled drinking. TFFFF

The following statements apply to drug dependence:

A. tolerance to the effects of the drug always develops
B. affected individuals usually experience a compulsion to take a drug
C. drug abuse is a form of drug dependence
D. physical withdrawal symptoms always occur upon abstinence
E. the term applies only to the abuse of drugs not generally available on prescription

Drug abuse is the persistent or sporadic use of a drug inconsistent with, or unrelated to, acceptable medical practice. **Drug dependence** has been defined by the World Health Organization as 'a state, psychic and sometimes also physical, resulting from the interaction between a living organism and a drug, characterised by behavioural and other responses that always include a compulsion to take a drug on a continuous or periodic basis in order to experience its psychic effects and sometimes to avoid the discomfort of its absence.' According to these definitions, not all cases of drug abuse are examples of drug dependence.

Tolerance to the effects of the drug and the development of physical withdrawal symptoms on abstinence are variable features depending on the drug(s) involved. Thus marked tolerance commonly develops to the effects of alcohol and opiates, but is less pronounced with barbiturates and minimal with amphetamines and LSD. Physical withdrawal symptoms do not occur with some drugs (such as the amphetamines) while others give rise to characteristic abstinence syndromes. Withdrawal from alcohol or barbiturates leads to acute brain syndromes, often complicated by epilepsy. Effects of opiate withdrawal include anxiety, irritability, excessive yawning, lachrymation, piloerection, dilated pupils and abdominal cramps. Benzodiazepines commonly give rise to withdrawal symptoms (see MCQ 121).

Dependence on more than one drug is common. Multiple dependence may occur at the same time, or dependence on particular drugs may succeed or alternate with each other.

The potential for dependence is recognised within an ever-increasing group of drugs including many which are among the most commonly prescribed drugs in medical practice, such as benzodiazepines, analgesics and anticholinergics. FTFFF

MCQ 79

The following statements apply to opiate dependence:

A. in Britain, the greatest prevalence is in Social Class 5
B. most addicts are psychiatrically ill
C. notification of suspected addicts to the Home Office is compulsory
D. in Britain the ultimate aim of treatment in all cases is maintenance on methadone
E. mortality among addicts is 2–3% per year

Prior to the 1960's opiate dependence was largely confined to those exposed therapeutically and to those in contact with the drugs professionally. Subsequently, drug abuse began to extend widely beyond these groups of people, and the incidence of opiate dependence increased rapidly. Since 1968 it has been compulsory for all doctors to notify the Home Office Central Register of suspected addicts. Despite this, Home Office statistics underestimate the prevalence of the problem—research studies in drug dependence units have demonstrated that each addict registered is in contact with at least one other addict not known to the Home Office. Among registered addicts, males outnumber females by a factor of four to one. Peak age of this population is in the second and third decades and there is a second peak in middle age. All social classes are represented equally among addicts in Britain, in contrast to the United States where dependence is associated with underprivilege and minority ethnic groups.

Both biological and psychosocial factors may play a part in opiate dependence and theories of aetiology are diverse and conjectural. Current practice emphasises a multifactorial approach to the problem.

Only a small proportion of addicts display frank psychiatric illness. In one research study, 55% of cases warranted a diagnosis of drug dependence alone. Some 5–10% were neurotic and only 1–3% schizophrenic. The remainder were considered to have abnormal personalities but no frank psychiatric illness.

The management of opiate dependence in Britain is undertaken largely in locally-based drug dependence clinics. In Britain, certain drugs (including heroin and cocaine) may be legally prescribed only by specially licensed doctors, who generally operate from such clinics. The patient is commenced on a reducing regime of opiate substitute. Methadone is commonly employed owing to its long half-life and the fact that it can be administered orally thus removing the need for continued intravenous injection. Only rarely are injectable opiates prescribed. More recently the technique of electrostimulation and the administration of clonidine have become alternatives to regimes of opiate withdrawal. Abstinence should be the aim of treatment, although some patients only manage to transfer to maintenance doses of methadone. However, the efficacy of such maintenance methadone regimes remains controversial.

In addition to treatment for physical withdrawal syndromes, the clinics offer counselling and social support to addicts and their families and in some cases day centre and inpatient detoxification facilities. Successful treatment depends largely on maintaining motivation.

Some 50% of individuals who engage in opiate abuse become physically dependent. Of those who become dependent 2–3% die each year. After five years, 25% are abstinent and after ten years some 40% have stopped. Reasons offered to explain this pattern include advancing age, the development of relationships with non-addicts and drastic changes in social circumstances. FFTFT

Adverse effects of cannabis include:

A. panic attacks
B. reduced spermatogenesis
C. precipitation or exacerbation of psychotic disorders
D. 'flashbacks'
E. physical dependence

The term 'cannabis' is used to describe a variety of natural and derived products from the plant 'Cannabis sativa'. A large number of names for these products exists throughout the world but essentially there are two kinds of material: the resinous exudate best known as 'hashish' and the chopped leaves and stalks known as 'grass' or 'marihuana'. These materials are usually smoked and occasionally mixed with food or drink. The active compound in both is tetrahydrocannabinol.

Effects of the drug include euphoria, relaxation and subjective feelings of well-being. Perceptual distortions may occur and rarely visual hallucinations. Physiological effects include lowered body temperature and increased appetite.

Psychological dependence may occur in some, while in others the drug may be discontinued with impunity. Physical dependence does not occur.

Severe adverse effects of cannabis are uncommon. Physical effects include reduced spermatogenesis and possible increase in tobacco-related diseases owing to the frequent use of tobacco in conjunction with cannabis. An increased incidence of foetal abnormalities has also been reported. Panic attacks may occur during intoxication, most commonly in naive users. Transient 'flashback' phenomena may occur in which the individual may experience the effects of intoxication well beyond the time the drug was taken. If LSD has also been abused cannabis intoxication may also provoke 'flashbacks' to the experience of LSD intoxication.

The relationship between cannabis abuse and functional psychosis is unclear. Acute psychoses have been reported in association with cannabis intoxication but it would appear that in a substantial proportion of such cases features of acute brain syndrome are also present. Subacute psychoses without the characteristic features of organic brain syndromes ★ have also been reported, but the causative role of cannabis has not been clearly established. Cannabis abuse may however exacerbate pre-existing schizophrenic illness.

An 'amotivational' syndrome characterised by apathy, reduced drive and lack of ambition has been described in Eastern and Caribbean studies, but other factors such as poor nutrition and lack of economic opportunity may contribute, and cannabis abuse has not clearly established as a cause of this syndrome. TTTTF

The following statements apply to solvent abuse among adolescents:

A. males considerably outnumber females
B. most abusers are psychiatrically disturbed
C. visual hallucinations are a recognised symptom of abuse
D. no serious physical complications of abuse have been reported
E. inpatient detoxification is normally required

No satisfactory data are available on the extent or precise characteristics of solvent abuse among adolescents, but the problem appears to be more common in deprived families living in inner urban areas. Males outnumber females among those affected by a factor of up to ten to one.

The agents abused are volatile hydrocarbons, of which the most common are proprietary brands of glue. Most agents contain toluene or acetone. A variety of methods of inhalation is used, the most dangerous of which include the use of polythene bags placed over the head to concentrate fumes and the direct spraying of aerosols into the mouth or nose. Effects include euphoria or exhilaration, although visual hallucinations may occur with more severe intoxication. These effects may be followed by a period of disorientation, blurred vision, ataxia and slurred speech.

The majority of adolescents abusing solvents do not suffer physical damage. Severe physical disorders and death have however been reported. Systematic complications may include haematological disorders such as eosinophilia and anaemia, renal damage, cardiac arrythmias and toluene encephalopathy. The use of more dangerous methods of inhalation (such as using a polythene bag to concentrate fumes) increases the risk of these physical complications and may lead to asphyxiation.

Adolescents who sniff glue commonly do so as part of a group activity, in which case the phenomenon can be seen as a means of expressing adolescent conflicts and rebellion. In most such cases there is no underlying psychiatric disturbance. Such abuse is usually transient and no physical complications or dependence develop. A smaller proportion of adolescents abuse solvents as a means of escape from the stress of disturbed family or environmental circumstances. For this latter group, abuse is generally a solitary activity. Here, there is a tendency to use the more dangerous methods of inhalation and for the abuse to persist.

Educating adolescents about solvent abuse is an important part of management. Adolescents require explanation of the risk of solvent abuse, and in particular the risks associated with the more dangerous methods of inhalation. Psychiatric referral is usually not required unless the abuse is severe, prolonged, associated with physical side-effects, or where a pattern of severe family disruption is seen to underlie the disorder. Hospital admission may occasionally be required for the management of physical complications or in order to break an entrenched pattern of severe abuse and dependence. TFTFF

Eating Disorders

MCQ 82

Anorexia nervosa is characterised by the following:

A. increased libido
B. amenorrhoea
C. bradycardia
D. avitaminosis
E. a relentless pursuit of thinness

Anorexia nervosa has three characteristic diagnostic features. The first is weight loss, usually in excess of 20% of the healthy weight. Secondly, an endocrine disturbance is present, consisting of amenorrhoea in the female and loss of libido in the male. Lastly, there is a characteristic psychopathology which includes a relentless pursuit of thinness, an apparent morbid fear of fatness and a distorted body image such that the individual overestimates her weight and size.

A proportion of patients induce vomiting as a means of losing weight and about one in three indulge in periodic 'binges' of high carbohydrate foods, usually followed by self-induced vomiting or purgation. Other methods of losing weight include vigorous and excessive exercise and abuse of diuretics or anorexic drugs. Mental symptoms include difficulties with concentration and a preoccupation with food and eating and body weight often to the extent of becoming all-consuming. The area of eating and weight control becomes a constant struggle, with the generation of guilt and hostility in the individual and the family. Surprisingly, the degree of depression is less than might be expected considering the degree of emaciation and disruption of family life and many patients are inappropriately optimistic and deny the seriousness of the condition. For this reason few patients agree readily to treatment.

A number of signs and symptoms appear secondary to the emaciation, including bradycardia, peripheral cyanosis, the growth of lanugo hair and tiredness and muscular weakness. Frequent self-induced vomiting may cause salivary gland enlargement or electrolyte disturbances but avitaminosis is rare. Demineralisation of the incisor teeth may occur due to erosion of tooth enamel by vomited gastric acid.

The condition is much commoner in females than males and usually begins in the late teens or early twenties, often in the setting of examinations or a proposed move away from the family. High-risk groups for the disorder include models and ballet dancers and it may be commoner among higher socioeconomic groups. FTTFT

The following statements are true regarding anorexia nervosa:

A. admission to hospital is mandatory
B. antidepressants are the mainstay of treatment
C. patients invariably recover within a short time of diagnosis
D. a short history predicts a better prognosis
E. some patients may go on to develop bulimia nervosa

In the acute phase of anorexia nervosa, treatment should be directed first at inducing weight gain. If the patient is of average build and weighs less than 35 kg, admission should be urgently considered. If the body weight is greater than 40 kg, especially if the weight loss has been gradual, outpatient treatment may be considered. This usually takes the form of a behavioural approach agreed with the patient and her family designed to induce weight gain. Usually this is overtly or covertly resisted and other techniques such as paradoxical ones may need to be employed. It is essential to form a working relationship with the patient and her family as a prelude to successful treatment. Once weight gain is underway, psychotherapy designed to support the patient and her family and also to understand the cause of the condition may be undertaken. There is little evidence that drugs alter the course of the illness. Antidepressants may be used if depression is prominent and antipsychotic drugs have been used during the phase of refeeding.

In cases of extreme emaciation, admission to hospital, preferably to a unit specialising in the treatment of eating disorders, should be arranged without delay. Sometimes the patient denies the necessity for treatment, and detention in hospital under the Mental Health Act ★ may be required. Fortunately, it is usually possible to avoid this by enlisting the assistance of other family members in persuading the patient to agree to voluntary treatment. Once in a specialised unit refeeding is usually relatively easy. Commonly, a behavioural approach is used, in which a contract is made with the patient such that by gaining the predetermined amount of weight in a given interval, she 'earns' reinforcement, such as greater freedom to move around the ward and visits from friends. Follow-up psychotherapy, either individually or in a family setting is mandatory. There is some evidence that younger patients do better with family therapy in that drop-out and relapse rates are lower.

The prognosis is best in patients with a short history. Disturbed premorbid personality, chronicity and onset later in life predict a poor prognosis. About one in three patients appears to recover completely after a single episode, while another half will remain disabled to some extent with relapses and remissions. Bulimia nervosa may develop. About 5% will die from suicide or other causes and a small number will develop other serious psychiatric illnesses such as bipolar affective disorder or rarely schizophrenia. The longer the period of follow-up the worse the prognosis appears, which suggests that the disorder is a serious one with complete long-term recovery being less common than has previously been assumed. FFFTT

MCQ 84

In bulimia nervosa:

A. patients are commonly grossly underweight
B. depressive symptoms are common
C. patients consume large quantities of high carbohydrate foods in one sitting
D. following 'binges' patients take steps to lose weight
E. self-induced vomiting and abuse of laxatives is common

Bulimia nervosa, a syndrome described by Russell in 1979, has three characteristic features. Patients suffer powerful and intractible urges to overeat. Secondly, they seek to avoid the 'fattening' effects of overeating by self-induced vomiting or laxative abuse or by severely restricting food intake between 'binges'. The third feature is the characteristic psychopathology, similar to that in anorexia nervosa, with a morbid fear of fatness and pursuit of thinness.

Although some anorexic patients may proceed to bulimia nervosa, many bulimics have never been grossly underweight. In contrast to anorexia nervosa, patients with bulimia nervosa may have a normal or even increased weight, but the commonest presentation is in the slightly underweight individual. Eating habits are grossly disorganised with severe restriction of calories and the erratic consumption of 'diet foods' punctuated by intermittent 'binges' of carbohydrate-rich foods. Huge quantities may be consumed at a sitting to be terminated by engorgement, lethargy and dysphoria and frequently followed by self-induced vomiting. Other measures to reduce weight include abuse of laxatives, often to an extreme extent, excessive exercise and abuse of appetite supressants or diuretics. Unlike anorexics, bulimic patients are often sexually active. Many have steady relationships and are living away from home. Depression and dysphoria are common, with patients focusing all their problems on their concerns with eating and weight.

Physical complications may occur, such as gastric dilatation, erosion of teeth, enlargement of salivary glands and abnominal pain secondary to laxative abuse. If vomiting is extreme, electrolyte imbalance, particularly hypokalaemia, may be present, and this may be relevant to sudden death which has been rarely described in these patients.

Like anorexia nervosa, this syndrome is much more common in females than males but occurs in a slightly older age group than anorexia. The condition appears to be common and most milder cases probably never reach medical attention. Prevalence rates of 1 in 200 have been found in high-risk groups such as female college students and less severe forms of the illness may be even more common. FTTTT

Bulimia nervosa:

A. may improve with antidepressant treatment
B. usually has an excellent prognosis
C. is usually managed by admitting the patient to hospital
D. has an unknown aetiology
E. is compatible with reasonably normal social and occupational functioning

Treatment should initially be directed at normalising the pattern of eating, for which behavioural techniques are often useful. Patients should be instructed to keep a written record of their diet and instructed to consume a normal mixed diet. Support and encouragement are necessary to allay fears of weight gain. Antidepressants may be prescribed if depression is prominent. As the eating pattern normalises and the frequency of binges and vomiting declines, exploration sometimes reveals conflicts which were hidden behind the eating problem which may now be addressed. Admission to hospital is rarely indicated, unless the eating pattern is so disrupted that change is impossible or there are severe physical complications.

The aetiology is unknown. Physiological, behavioural and dynamic explanations have been proposed but none explains the peculiar self-destructive cycle which characterises this disorder.

The outcome of the bulimia nervosa is not clearly understood. Russell described an invariably poor outcome but his cases were probably unusually severe. Subsequent authors have described a much more favourable outcome, with good results from behavioural, cognitive or pharmacological treatments or a combination of these. There may be a good response to tricyclic or monoamine oxidase inhibitor antidepressants alone, at least in the short term. It may be that there are two populations of bulimics, one with a poor prognosis and one with a relatively good outcome. The former may be cases with a long history of bulimia, or a previous history of anorexia nervosa, while the latter seem to be patients with a good social and occupational adjustment and high motivation for change. TFFTT

Suicide and Deliberate Self-harm

MCQ 86

The following statements regarding completed suicide are true:

A. predominantly Protestant countries record higher rates than countries which are predominantly Catholic
B. it is associated with physical illness
C. it is associated with psychiatric disturbance
D. it is more common among women than men
E. the rate peaks in spring

Precise suicide rates are very difficult to determine. There is evidence that official statistics underestimate suicide rates, and interpretations of what constitutes 'suicide' may differ considerably, particularly from one country to another. This partly accounts for the variation between countries of reported rates of suicide. Although it was suggested in the past that Protestant countries had higher suicide rates than Catholic ones, this is not confirmed by official statistics. For example, both Austria and Italy are predominantly Catholic. The suicide rate in Austria is amongst the highest in Europe, that in Italy one of the lowest.

Suicide rates are higher for men than for women (although this sex difference is becoming less marked) and rise with increasing age. Suicide is more common among the divorced, the widowed and single people than those who are married. Social isolation is an important factor. Suicides are more frequent in areas of high unemployment. During both World Wars, the suicide rate in Britain dropped dramatically—among the factors suggested to account for this observation is the drop in unemployment during wartime.

The rates of suicide are not uniform throughout the year. In Britain and other northern hemisphere countries, the incidence of suicide peaks in April–June. The same pattern, with a peak incidence in spring and early summer, is found in southern hemisphere countries.

Many of those people who successfully commit suicide have a past history of psychiatric illness, and researchers have suggested that 90% or more were psychiatrically ill at the time they killed themselves. However, these figures are difficult to substantiate, because they obviously rely to some degree on retrospective data.

Another important factor associated with suicide is physical illness. This is present in one third or more of those who kill themselves—in this population, physical illness and depression commonly occur together. FTTFT

The following statements apply to people who have committed suicide:

A. in most cases, they had not mentioned their suicidal ideas to their general practitioner or other people involved with them
B. the most common method chosen is an overdose with prescribed drugs
C. violent methods of suicide, e.g. hanging, are as frequent among women as among men
D. 5–10% of cases will have shown no evidence shortly before death of psychiatric illness
E. 10% or more will have previously attempted suicide

Most of those who commit suicide were psychiatrically ill (see MCQ 88) although a small minority of this group will have shown no evidence of psychiatric disturbance (it is worth remembering, however, that studies of suicide have been retrospective and relevant information may therefore be incomplete). In most cases, the person will have declared his/her suicidal intent to friends or professionals. In one well-known study of suicides in one part of England, one-third of the sample made unequivocal statements of suicidal intent (this is likely to be an underestimate of the real frequency) and more than half offered hints in this direction. Two-thirds of this sample had visited a doctor in the month before killing themselves. 80% of the whole sample were receiving psychotropic medication.

It has been estimated that a previous episode of deliberate self-harm increases the risk of suicide 100-fold compared with the general population. Estimates of the percentage of people with a history of deliberate self-harm who subsequently kill themselves vary between 10% and over 40%.

Approximately 90% of suicides follow self-poisoning with drugs. Since the 1960's, this has replaced gassing as the most common method of suicide. The observed decline in the use of gas coincided with the switch to natural gas, which is not as noxious as the coal gas used before this time. More violent methods, such as hanging, jumping and the use of guns, are far less common and have altered little in frequency over the years. Among those who use such violent means of suicide, males are much more common than females.

The extent to which a particular agent is available as a means of suicide undoubtedly affects the relative frequency of suicides by that method—the introduction of natural gas in Britain and other parts of Europe demonstrated this well. Rather more controversial is the suggestion that easier access to an effective means of suicide increases the overall suicide rate. Some researchers have described a positive correlation between total prescriptions of psychotropic drugs and frequency of hospital admissions for deliberate self-harm. However, such an association does not necessarily imply a causal connection. In any case, it is important to remember that while prescriptions for psychotropic drugs have been rising, the rate of completed suicides (as opposed to episodes of non-fatal self-poisoning) has been falling. Thus it is unlikely that increasing access to an effective method of suicide will dramatically affect the overall suicide rate. FTFTF

Which of the following are recognised as factors contributing to suicide risk?

A. history of depression or alcohol abuse
B. epilepsy
C. history of obsessional neurosis
D. being elderly
E. being socially isolated

Suicide risk factors are usually considered in terms of the particular features which distinguish completed suicides, as a group, from the general population from which they are drawn.

Suicide is more common among men than women (MCQ 86). For both sexes, the suicide rate rises with increasing age, but this age effect is more pronounced for men than for women. Social isolation is another factor— suicide is more common among the divorced and widowed than among those who are married.

A number of psychiatric illnesses are associated with a higher than expected suicide rate, most notably affective disorder and alcoholism. More than half of those who commit suicide warranted a diagnosis of depression at the time of death. Conversely, it has been estimated that one in eight people who have at some time suffered from a severe depressive illness will eventually kill themselves. Other psychiatric diagnoses associated with an increased risk of suicide include organic brain syndromes, schizophrenia and drug addiction. An increased suicide rate is not found in *all* psychiatric disorders. Among people with obsessional neurosis, for example, the suicide rate is lower than expected.

Physical illness, particularly when chronic, is associated with a higher than average suicide rate (MCQ 86). Patients with epilepsy have a suicide rate approximately five times that of the general population. This risk is even greater when patients with temporal lobe epilepsy are considered alone. Other chronic illnesses are similarly associated with a high suicide rate; for example, it has been suggested that patients on renal dialysis have a suicide rate 400 times that of the general population. However, in this group of patients as in many others with chronic illness, it is non-compliance with medical treatment which leads to death in many cases. Such non-compliance is probably attributed to suicidal intent more frequently than it deserves.

A history of previous overdoses or other attempts at deliberate self-harm is also associated with an increased risk of suicide.

Suicide risk alone gives no direct information about suicide **intent** ★. TTFTT

Which of the following statements are true of deliberate self-harm (attempted suicide)?

A. it is most common in middle-aged females
B. among young adults, it is at least ten times more frequent than completed suicide
C. it constitutes 10% or more of acute medical admissions in the adult age group below 65 years
D. it is associated with major depression in more than 60% of cases
E. it is commonly associated with physical illness

Non-fatal deliberate self-harm (also known as parasuicide or attempted suicide) currently constitutes some 12% of acute medical admissions in England and Wales. Among cases of deliberate self-harm, females greatly outnumber males. Most frequent among young adults, its incidence (unlike that of completed suicide) declines with age. In the age group 15–24 years, cases of deliberate self-harm outnumber suicides by 400 to one for females, 20 to one for males.

The majority of episodes of deliberate self-harm are impulsive gestures which result from interpersonal difficulties, such as an argument with a boy- or girlfriend. In most cases, there is no evidence of serious physical or psychiatric illness, although there will often be evidence of a depressive reaction on admission to hospital. Unlike a depressive illness, such depressive reactions are transient and usually resolve spontaneously, without the need for specific psychiatric intervention. However, it is important to recognise and offer appropriate psychiatric treatment to the minority of patients who are clinically depressed.

In all these features, patients admitted for deliberate self-harm contrast with those who successfully commit suicide (see MCQ 88). Bearing in mind that a history of deliberate self-harm increases the likelihood of subsequent suicide (MCQ 87), the considerable differences between these two groups may at first seem surprising. However, it must be remembered that overall admissions for deliberate self-harm greatly outnumber completed suicides. Most people admitted with deliberate self-harm will *not* go on to commit suicide, and the majority of completed suicides will have no previous history of deliberate self-harm. FTTFF

In the assessment of a patient admitted after a deliberate overdose of drugs, the following are indicators of high suicidal intent:

A. having taken more than one type of drug
B. having made plans before the overdose to avoid discovery
C. the patient expresses ambivalence about whether or not he/she still wishes to die
D. a history of having taken previous overdoses
E. not having taken alcohol beforehand

It is important to consider separately suicide **intent** and suicide **risk** (the latter is considered in more detail in MCQ 88). Both of these need to be assessed carefully as part of the management of the suicidally inclined. The distinction is often unclear, but attempting to make it can help in the assessment of suicidal patients. The fact that someone falls into a high-risk group for suicide does not itself imply that suicide is his/her intention. Although up to one in five people with a history of severe affective illness will eventually kill themselves, this does not mean that all depressed patients show suicidal intent. Similarly, a history of previous deliberate self-harm makes further similar episodes more likely but does not relate directly to suicidal intent.

Several factors are important in the assessment of suicidal intent. First, what preparations did the person make? If the overdose was impulsive, this suggests a lower degree of intent than if the person had planned it carefully for weeks, saving up tablets deliberately, for example. The person could have settled all his affairs and made out a will. Whether or not someone tells others of his suicidal intent is not particularly helpful in assessment; many people who take overdoses without the intention of committing suicide do this, but so do a significant proportion of people who do subsequently commit suicide.

The second factor concerns the overdose itself. Was the person alone at the time of the overdose (this suggests greater suicidal intent)? What precautions were taken against discovery (such as waiting until everyone else was out, locking doors, etc.)? How did he/she get into hospital? Did the patient summon help, or did someone else discover what had happened? Consumption of alcohol before an overdose is common; this does not really offer much help in assessing suicidal intent. The patient's own account is very important here. Some patients will admit that they did not intend to kill themselves but wished to go to sleep for a long time in the hope of awakening with their problems solved. The patient's feelings should be elicited about having survived the overdose; some will be relieved, others angry that they are still alive. Ambivalence is common.

The potential lethality of the overdose is another vital factor. Would the patient have died without medical intervention? The patient's own statement of lethality must also be considered. An elderly man who takes a handful of iron tablets might well have believed them to be enough to kill him. Taking more than one type of drug is not in itself an indication of serious suicidal intent. Attempts to commit suicide by 'violent' means such as hanging are generally considered to imply high suicidal intent. FTFFF

Sexual Function and its Abnormalities

MCQ 91

Which of the following statements about the human sexual response are true?

A. the parasympathetic sacral outflow (S2,3,4) is thought to be involved in the mediation of penile erection
B. the mechanism of penile erection involves dilation of the arterial vasculature and closure of venous valves
C. the excitement phase of the female sexual response immediately precedes the orgasm phase
D. the refractory period occurs equally in both males and females
E. anxiety can be a powerful inhibitor of arousal

The sexual response in both males and females is divided into four phases. First, the **excitement phase** is accompanied by early signs of sexual arousal including erection in males and vaginal lubrication in females. This is followed by the **plateau phase**, a stage during which the increase of sexual arousal levels off. After a variable amount of time, the **orgasm phase** follows, during which ejaculation occurs in the male and pubo-coccygeus muscular contraction occurs in the female. The last phase is **resolution** when the anatomical and physiological changes that have occurred return to normal. In males there is a **refractory period** during which further ejaculation is not possible. A refractory period does not generally occur in females.

The neural mechanism of erection is not clearly understood. Erection involves dilation of arterioles and closure of venous valves. The arteriolar dilation is probably controlled by the parasympathetic supply carried in the pelvic nerves. However, the sympathetic supply from the lumbar outflow probably has a role, and the two systems may work synergistically in the mediation of both the erectile and ejaculatory responses.

Anxiety can be a powerful inhibitor of arousal, and is associated with most of the specific sexual dysfunctions. Traditionally, reduction of anxiety associated with sexual activity has been an important component of behaviour therapy programmes for sexual problems (see MCQ 94). TTFFT

Which of the following statements about sexual dysfunction are true?

A. premature ejaculation is the most common problem among males who present to sexual dysfunction clinics

B. vaginismus is the most common problem among females who present to sexual dysfunction clinics

C. in surveys of the general population, the most common sexual problem reported by women is impaired sexual interest

D. surveys of the general population reveal that at least 1 in 10 females never experiences orgasm

E. surveys of the general population suggest that erectile dysfunction occurs in less than 10% of men but the proportion increases with age.

Erectile dysfunction is the commonest problem among males presenting at sexual dysfunction clinics (40–60%) followed by premature ejaculation (about 20%) and retarded ejaculation (less than 10%). Impaired sexual interest is the commonest problem in females (about 50%) presenting at sexual dysfunction clinics, followed by orgasmic dysfunction (about 20%), vaginismus (less than 20%) and dyspareunia (less than 5%).

In surveys of the general population, erectile impotence occurs in less than 10% of males but the proportion increases with age. Premature ejaculation is reported by at least one-third of males. Such surveys also reveal primary anorgasmia as a problem in at least 10% of women. These sexual dysfunctions are not always associated with sexual dissatisfaction, that is, they are not necessarily considered to be problems by those experiencing them. Further, analysis of the prevalence of sexual dysfunctions in these terms fails to take into account the combination of different types of dysfunction which occur in individuals, and within couples. For example, in couples presenting with sexual dysfunctions, impairment of sexual interest in the female and premature ejaculation in the male are commonly associated. FFTTT

MCQ 93

Regarding sexual dysfunction:

A. erectile dysfunction and reduced sexual interest are very common in chronic alcoholism
B. erectile dysfunction occurs in up to 50% of men with diabetes mellitus
C. an individual's previous level of sexual interest and activity is usually preserved following myocardial infarction
D. increased sexual interest is a common problem in patients with epilepsy, particularly temporal lobe epilepsy
E. episiotomy often causes dyspareunia which may be persistent in some cases

Although psychological factors are the commonest cause of sexual dysfunction, physical illness, surgery and drug treatment can affect sexual functioning. In many cases, a combination of psychological and physical factors are important.

Endocrine disorders such as diabetes mellitus, Cushing's syndrome and adrenal insufficiency can be associated within impaired sexual interest, erectile dysfunction and orgasmic problems. Erectile dysfunction is common with hyperthyroidism, while hypothyroidism is associated in the majority of cases (male and female) with impaired sexual interest. Pituitary disease is also the cause of sexual problems: hyperprolactinaemia causes erectile dysfunction while hypopituitarism is associated with erectile and ejaculatory problems, orgasmic dysfunction, and reduced sexual interest in both sexes. Low sexual interest commonly occurs in patients with epilepsy, especially temporal lobe epilepsy.

Patients with hypertension have an increased prevalence of erectile dysfunction and ejaculatory failure, but these may be largely effects of antihypertensive medication. Following myocardial infarction there is a steady decline in sexual interest and activity, with erectile impotence occurring in a substantial proportion of patients. This outcome may be partly the result of fear of angina or further infarction, and possibly a lack of appropriate advice from doctors. These sexual problems are commoner in older patients.

A very high proportion of men and women with renal failure have sexual problems, mainly reduced sexual interest, erectile dysfunction and difficulty achieving orgasm. Renal dialysis is seldom beneficial in this regard, and the sexual difficulties may continue after renal transplantation.

Gynaecological surgical procedures can cause sexual problems. Episiotomy often leads to dyspareunia and this may be long-lasting in a small proportion of cases. Hysterectomy has variable effects on sexuality. Specific sexual dysfunctions are uncommon after the procedure but women who have a stong personal investment in their fertility may experience problems. More usually, patients show a significant improvement in both their enjoyment and the frequency of sexual intercourse after the hysterectomy. TTFFT

Which of the following techniques may be used in a behavioural programme for sexual problems?

A. the use of lubrication such as body lotion or K-Y jelly
B. the use of a vibrator for persistent orgasmic dysfunction
C. waxing and waning of erections for erectile dysfunction
D. graded vaginal dilators for dyspareunia
E. the bridge manoeuvre for retarded ejaculation

A behavioural programme for sexual problems is essentially a desensitisation procedure ★, and the couple receive regular 'homework' assignments incorporating graded tasks. In addition to the behavioural components of therapy, educating the partners about their own and each other's sexual responses is important. Also, the partners are encouraged to discuss and help each other understand their sexual relationship.

The behavioural programme usually begins with the couple being encouraged to discover how to give each other sexual enjoyment through caressing one another (this is termed 'the sensate focus') but genital contact is initially banned. Progressively, the graded homework exercises progress to genital contact and stimulation. The use of body lotion and K-Y jelly is often suggested by the therapist at this stage. The programme proceeds to 'vaginal containment', often employing the female superior position for intercourse. This aims to minimise the anxiety some couples have about sexual intercourse. The couple then progress to vaginal containment with movement.

Orgasmic dysfunction often responds to an additional masturbation-training programme for the female partner, and a vibrator is often successfully employed, temporarily, if the problem initially fails to improve. Once orgasm is occurring regularly during genital sensate focus, a 'bridge manoeuvre' can be adopted to help the woman reach orgasm during sexual intercourse. The woman receives clitoral stimulation either by herself or her partner, during vaginal containment.

For women with vaginismus, persuading the patient to insert the tip of her finger into the vaginal entrance is the first step in treatment, coupled with encouragement to talk about her anxieties regarding vaginal penetration. Subsequently, her partner should attempt penetration with one or more fingers. Graded vaginal dilators can be used if the patient experiences difficulty moving from finger to penile penetration. However, this is not part of a behavioural programme.

For erectile problems, one additional technique is to allow the male's erection to subside and return repeatedly during the genital sensate focus stage. This manoeuvre is designed to reassure the man who may be fearful that, once lost, his erection will not be easily regained. TTTFF

MCQ 95

Premature ejaculation

A. was defined by Masters and Johnson as ejaculation by the male partner before the female partner reached orgasm on at least half the occasions the couple had sexual intercourse
B. can be effectively treated using Seman's technique
C. has a reported cure rate about 40%
D. is commoner in men over 40 years of age
E. is a recognised side-effect of monoamine oxidase inhibitors

Premature ejaculation is a disorder in which the individual is unable to exert voluntary control over the ejaculatory reflex so that, following sexual arousal, orgasm occurs too quickly. The condition has also been variously defined as ejaculation occurring before penetration, less than two minutes after penetration, or upon fewer than 10 pelvic thrusts. Masters and Johnson considered the condition to be present if the male reached orgasm during intercourse before the female on more than 50% of occasions.

Premature ejaculation tends to be commoner in younger men. The condition responds well to behavioural psychotherapy techniques along the lines pioneered by Masters and Johnson, who claimed improvement with treatment in over 90% of cases. Equivalent figures reported in more recent studies vary from 55% to over 80%. Specifically, the 'squeeze' technique (or Seman's 'stop and start' technique which is very similar) can be effective in the context of a behavioural sex therapy programme. In the squeeze technique, the man gains an erection and either masturbates himself or is masturbated by his partner. Immediately before ejaculation his partner applies the squeeze technique by firmly placing her thumb on the frenulum and her first two fingers on either side of the coronal sulcus. The penis is squeezed for a few seconds. The man will lose his desire to ejaculate and usually experiences partial loss of the erection. The procedure is repeated and allows the man gradually to learn to control his ejaculatory response.

Monoamine oxidase inhibitors have been reported to cause erectile problems and possibly retrograde ejaculation but not premature ejaculation. Indeed, they have been used in a few uncontrolled studies as a treatment for premature ejaculation, although there is no convincing evidence that they can produce any sustained benefit in this condition. TTFFF

Retrograde ejaculation:

A. is a side-effect of antipsychotic drugs
B. can produce suprapubic pain
C. can occur as a complication of prostatectomy
D. usually responds to behaviour therapy
E. can produce 'white urine'

This is a condition is which semen is discharged into the bladder rather than through the anterior urethra due to inadequate closure of the internal sphincter. There may be an associated awareness of loss of ejaculate volume and occasionally suprapubic pain. Cloudy, post-orgasmic urine may be reported due to the presence of ejaculate in the bladder. The condition is a relatively common side-effect of antipsychotic drugs, particularly thioridazine. One study found that a third of patients taking this drug suffered from retrograde ejaculation. The problem may be related to the adrenergic blocking action, and possibly the anticholinergic effects, of antipsychotic drugs. Although the mechanism is unclear, it could involve interference with bladder neck closure and seminal emission but leave intact anterograde ejaculation and the associated sensations. The condition may also occur as a complication of prostatectomy, or following spinal injury. TTTFT

Regarding sexual deviance:

A. the most common fetishes are articles of clothing
B. transexualism is a type of transvestism
C. gynaecomastia is a potentially irreversible side-effect of cyproterone acetate, an antiandrogen used to control unwanted sexual desire
D. paedophiles are usually uninterested and/or unsuccessful in sexual relationships with other adults
E. the majority of indecent exposers are charged with the offence on repeated occasions

Fetishism is the use of an inanimate object to attain sexual arousal. The most common fetishes are articles of female attire, shoes and rubber clothing. Specific conditioning of the sexual response to the particular stimulus is thought to be relevant to the genesis of this condition and such a deviation of the normal sexual development seems to be almost exclusively a male susceptibility.

Transsexualism is a disorder of gender identity: transsexuals believe they belong to the opposite sex despite the evidence of their anatomy. Both male and female transsexuals have a strong desire to change their physical appearance so that it is consistent with their psychological gender. To this end, they will often seek medical help. Gender reassignment involves hormone administration and surgery, and stringent criteria are applied before such treatments are employed.

Transvestism involves repeatedly dressing in clothes of the opposite sex (cross-dressing). Often, cross-dressing is accompanied by sexual excitement (in other words, the clothes worn are fetish objects) although it may also have a function to relieve anxiety. Although some transvestites are homosexuals, many are married, and in some cases the spouse is aware of the cross-dressing. Unlike transsexuals, transvestites do not believe they belong to the opposite sex and do not seek gender reassignment. Transsexuals also differ from transvestites in that transsexuals do not normally become sexually aroused by crossdressing.

Exhibitionism refers to intentional but inappropriate display of the genitalia, invariably by a man to a woman or girl. In most cases, the exposer has an erect penis and masturbates during or after the act which he finds sexually exciting. The majority of men charged with indecent exposure of this kind do not re-offend.

A **paedophile** is an adult who is sexually attracted to pre-pubertal children, usually with a particular preference for either male or female children. This deviant sexual predilection is socially and legally proscribed, although the majority of practising paedophiles are never identified or convicted. Most paedophiles have experienced difficulties in developing and maintaining stable relationships, especially sexual relationships, with other mature adults.

Drugs are sometimes used in individuals with deviant sexual interest to reduce the intensity of the sexual drive, and thus curb the antisocial sexual behaviour. However, these antilibidinal drugs fail to modify the choice of sexual object or the mode of sexual behaviour, and may have unpleasant side-effects. For example, oestrogens are associated with nausea and feminising effects, while with cyproterone acetate, an antiandrogen, there is a risk of potentially irreversible gynaecomastia. In view of such adverse effects, and the context in which these drugs are usually prescribed, it is prudent to administer them only with the written consent of the patient. TFTTF

Child Psychiatry and Mental Handicap

Regarding psychiatric disorders in children:

A. they may be adequately classified in terms of clinical syndromes, as in psychiatric disorders affecting adults
B. they are more common in children with physical illness affecting the central nervous system than with other types of physical illness
C. conduct disorders are equally common in girls and boys
D. emotional disorders are more common in boys than girls
E. their prevalence is inversely related to intelligence

A major distinction between classification of adult psychiatric disorders and those which occur in childhood is that the latter occur in the context of a child's development. Behaviour which may be characteristic of one stage of development may be atypical at other stages—good examples are enuresis ★ and encopresis (faecal soiling). What makes this picture even more complex is that development itself is not a unitary concept—it includes not only physical (biological) growth and maturation but also emotional, cognitive and social dimensions (MCQ 99). Also, the dependence of children on their families or on other adults makes them particularly vulnerable to the adverse effects of family discord, understimulation, and so on. For these reasons, classification of psychiatric disorders in childhood is even less successful than in adults if it relies only on clinical symptom clusters or syndromes (MCQ 2).

With this proviso, it it possible to define two main types of psychiatric problem in childhood—**conduct disorders** and **emotional disorders**. Emotional disorders include symptoms like fear, anxiety, misery and somatic complaints. Conduct disorders include disobedience, aggression, disruptiveness and destructiveness. Conduct disorders may be further subdivided into **socialised** and **unsocialised** types, depending on whether the child manifests the disturbance as part of a peer group or when alone. Socialised conduct disorders, such as might result from being a member of a 'gang', often involve behaviour which is seen as normal within a particular subcultural group.

The prevalence of psychiatric disturbance among 10–11 year olds varies from 5–20%, being lower in rural areas than in inner cities. Boys are more commonly affected than girls. Most types of disturbance are also more common in boys than girls, with the exception of emotional disorders, which are equally common in both sexes. A wide variety of psychiatric problems are more common among children of lower intelligence than those with higher IQ. Psychiatric disturbance is twice as common in children with a physical disorder not involving the brain (like asthma) and five times more likely if a brain disorder exists (like epilepsy and/or brain damage). FTFFT

Which of the following can be regarded as normal or expected for the age stated?

A. selective attachment to a parent at 7 months
B. predominantly reciprocal play with other children at 12 months
C. active searching for toys which have been hidden in the child's presence at 10 months
D. smiling selectively at particular faces at 3 months
E. playing in groups according to group rules at 5 years

Adequate assessment of a child's emotional or cognitive state depends very much on knowing what to expect of a child of this age. Abnormalities may either reflect developmental delay or immaturity, or may be specific. An example of the latter type of abnormality is **specific reading retardation**. This presents with problems in reading and writing (and possibly also other aspects of language). Other intellectual abilities are at the level expected for the child's age. The condition is more common in boys than girls, and is associated in some cases with minor neurological abnormalities.

Although the neonate is equipped to make emotional responses, these develop over time in their selectivity and reciprocity. Initially, a baby will smile at eye-like dots as well as faces, but by the age of 5 months, infants will respond to particular facial expressions. Only later (at about 7 months of age) do they selectively recognise particular faces. As with other aspects of development, this progression depends very much on the infant's environment and stimulation. Blindness in the infant commonly results in delaying smiling.

Attachment—the persistent selective bonding of the infant with an adult, most commonly a parent (usually its mother, but possibly its father)—develops in the first year. It tends to become manifest at about 7 months of age, and is heralded by specific behaviours like protest at separation. Before this age, infants are much less selective about adults, and are usually happy to be with a stranger as with a parent. By the end of the first year also, the infant is beginning to make functional use of objects (like toys).

Play is initially 'object-centred'—at 6–8 months of age, infants will commonly ignore their peers most of the time while playing. In the second year, play becomes more sociable, but initially involves doing things in parallel with other children. By the age of 3 years, there is usually evidence of active cooperative play, and by 5 years children will usually play within a group of their peers, according to group rules.

The neonate has a very rudimentary concept of 'self' and 'other'. At 3 months, the infant will follow its mother with its eyes and continue to stare at the point where mother was last seen (like the door). Before the age of about 10 months, the infant will consider that any object obscured from view has 'disappeared'. After this time, he is likely to seek actively a hidden object in a particular place, where it was first hidden and found. Some months later (at about 18 months old), when the capacity for symbolic thought has begun to develop, the child will be able to comprehend that the object still exists but is hidden somewhere and will be able to imagine a number of places where the object might be hidden. TFTFT

School refusal:

A. is not commonly associated with conduct disorder
B. most commonly presents at the age of 11 years
C. may be distinguished from truancy by the fact that the child's whereabouts are usually known to its parents
D. is associated with antisocial behaviour
E. like truancy, is associated with poor academic performance

School refusal refers to the fearful inability to attend school. It is sometimes described as **school phobia**. It has three peaks of prevalence—at or shortly after entry to school for the first time (age 5–7 years), at the time of changing schools (age 11) and at 14 years or older. The most common age at presentation is 11 years. In the youngest of these groups, it is commonly associated with anxiety about leaving parents (separation anxiety). Older children may either have specific fears relating to attending school (such as travelling, assemblies or being bullied) or suffer from other disturbances such as depression. Sometimes, school refusal may present with predominantly somatic symptoms, like abdominal pains, vague malaise or headaches.

School refusal must be distinguished from **truancy**, which is wilful and unjustifiable absence from school, initiated by the child himself. In the case of school refusal, the child's whereabouts are usually known to its parents (school refusers often remain at home). By contrast, truants do not usually remain at home when they are not at school—they may associate outside school with other children who are truanting. School refusal is not associated with poor academic performance or disruptive behaviour at school, although these are features of truancy. Other psychiatric problems associated with school refusal include anxiety and depression—conduct disorder and antisocial behaviour are more commonly found among those children who truant.

The initial step in management is recognition, which may be difficult, especially when the presentation is somatic (such as with recurrent 'tummy aches'). As with other childhood problems, assessment needs to include not only the child but also its parents and the family circumstances. Having established the nature of the difficulty, the main aim is to return the child to school as soon as possible. Especially when the problem presents acutely, this can be done successfully by involving parents, the school and the child in setting a specific date for the child to return to school and encouraging everyone involved to be consistent in carrying out this plan. When the problem is more longstanding, a behavioural programme involving a graded return to school (a form of systematic desensitisation ★) is often successful. TTTFF

Enuresis:

A. affects approximately 10% of children aged 10 years in Britain
B. when secondary at age 12 years is almost always due to psychological causes
C. is more common in larger families
D. is more common among children who have first-degree relatives who were or are also enuretic
E. may be cured in most cases using clomipramine

Enuresis (bedwetting) may be **primary** (in which case the child has never been dry) or **secondary** (when the child has become dry at night but subsequently resumes bedwetting). Bedwetting affects approximately 10% of 10 year olds, and 1% of 18 year olds. The condition is more common in boys than in girls. It is also associated with large families and other types of social adversity, like family discord or institutional upbringing. There is also a genetic component to the condition—there is a history of enuresis in a first-degree relative in the majority of cases and the concordance of enuresis among monozygotic twins is greater than that in dizygotic twins (see MCQ 10).

Enuresis, whether primary or secondary, may be due at any age to causes other than psychological ones. Assessment of a case of enuresis must include physical examination and appropriate investigations. Enuresis may be due to urinary tract infection or glycosuria. There may be structural or functional abnormalities in the bladder or another part of the urogenital tract. A neurological disorder may be present, although one which is severe enough to affect bladder function will usually also interfere with walking. Attention needs to be focused not only on the child but also the family and home circumstances. Wetting during the day as well as at night should arouse particular suspicion of urinary tract infections or other physical causes, although daytime wetting may sometimes be caused predominantly by psychological factors (for example, when a child is afraid to use the toilet at school).

Treatment begins with an adequate baseline assessment of the problem. This can be done by getting the child and parents to collaborate in completing a 'star chart', recording nights on which the child has been dry. Bedwetting may be considerably improved using tricyclic antidepressants like clomipramine, but in most cases, enuresis returns when the drug is discontinued. Thus this is usually not the treatment of choice. Behavioural techniques are most commonly used in treatment, notably the 'bell and pad' method, which is successful in the majority of cases. In this technique, a pad linked to a buzzer and a battery, is placed under the bedsheet. When the pad becomes wet as the child begins to urinate, this completes the electrical circuit, causing the buzzer to sound. The child is thus awoken and empties his bladder using a bedside pot. TFTTF

MCQ 102

Conduct disorders in childhood:

A. are associated with reading difficulties
B. are a type of delinquency
C. generally have a good prognosis
D. have been related in research studies to discord between parents
E. show a favourable response to small doses of haloperidol in approximately 20% of cases

Conduct disorders involve behaviour which is not only excessive (after taking the child's age into account) but which also impairs the child's development and/or causes the child to suffer. Conduct disorders are much more common in boys than girls, and may occur at any age, although they are more common during the preschool years and at the start of adolescence than at other times. Conduct disorders are associated with family or social disruption, organic brain dysfunction, larger families and lower intelligence. There is also an association with reading difficulties at school. However, the relative importance of these and other factors is difficult to ascertain. For example, some studies have reported an inverse relationship between prevalence of conduct disorder and parental social class. However, lower social class children are also more likely than others to have low IQ's and also to experience reading difficulties.

Conduct disorders must be distinguished from **delinquency**. A juvenile delinquent is a child who breaks the law. Delinquency is thus not a psychiatric diagnosis, but a legal definition. There is some overlap between delinquency and conduct disorders—delinquents who become recidivists (persistent offenders) are more likely than others to have a history of conduct disorder. However, many children with conduct disorders do not get into trouble with the law and most of those convicted of a first offence have no history of conduct disorder. In any case, there are many more delinquents than there are children with conduct disorders.

Management of children with conduct disorders is difficult. Depending on the individual case, the main focus for intervention will be the child himself, the family or the classroom (or possibly a combination of these). There is no evidence that antipsychotic drugs (or any other drugs) are effective.

The prognosis is generally unfavourable, particularly when conduct disturbance is associated with truancy. In boys, conduct disorders are linked with personality disorder in adulthood. One American study of boys referred to a child guidance clinic who showed seriously antisocial behaviour found after a 30-year follow-up that half of them persisted in showing antisocial behaviour (but see also MCQ 11). TFFTF

Regarding child abuse:

A. severe physical abuse is associated with a mortality rate of approximately 10%
B. sexual assault commonly involves physical attack
C. the risk of repetition when a child has already been physically abused is 60%
D. it is more common in families with parents who were themselves abused as children than in other families
E. it is significantly associated with psychiatric disorder in one or both parents

Child abuse refers to the inflicting of harm on, or neglect of, a child by those responsible for its care. Abuse may be physical, emotional or sexual and may also involve neglect. Although it may be easy to recognise abuse in extreme cases, it is sometimes difficult to define accurately what constitutes abuse—this depends on social and other norms which may vary considerably over time and also from place to place. This is particularly so for neglect. Because of this, and also the probably low detection rate and underreporting of cases, the prevalence of child abuse is difficult to determine.

Risk factors in the child include being the youngest child, having a mental or physical handicap, being separated from mother during the neonatal period, and resulting from an unwanted pregnancy. Features of the parents which point to a greater risk of child abuse include being a single parent, being young, and having been abused as a child. Psychiatric illness is not especially common among the parents of abused children. In addition to risk factors attributable to the child or to its parents, there are others associated with the family situation. These include social isolation, a large family and current stress (such as domestic friction or severe financial difficulties).

Physical abuse is much more common in children whose elder siblings have been abused. Especially when severe, it carries a grave prognosis. There is a mortality rate of approximately 10% associated with severe physical abuse, and a 60% risk of repeated non-accidental injury. There is also a significant long-term morbidity, both emotional and physical.

Incest and other forms of sexual abuse most commonly involve fathers or stepfathers and their daughters. Physical violence or extreme coercion are uncommon as a prelude to incest, but pressure may be brought on the child not to reveal the abuse. Sometimes, the other parent is aware of what is happening but colludes through non-disclosure. The abuse may go on for some years, commonly escalating from relatively minor acts of indecency to more overt sexual acts. Sexual abuse is associated with a high rate of emotional and behavioural disturbance both at the time of the abuse and often continuing into adulthood.

The recognition of child abuse may be difficult, but rests initially on maintaining a high index of suspicion. The main focus of management is to protect the interests of the child. Separating the child from its parents is one option, although there are some circumstances in which this is likely to do more harm than good and this decision should thus not be taken lightly. If the parents refuse to allow the child to leave the home, this may be done without the parents' consent using a Place of Safety Order. This is an order applied for by a social worker, on the basis of evidence gathered by all the professionals involved, and granted by a magistrate. In the longer term, management usually involves a case conference of professionals involved in the particular case, to assess the circumstances of the abuse, risks of recurrence, options for further management, and so on. If necessary, the child's name may be placed on the local authority 'at risk' register. A Care Order may also be sought by the social worker from the Juvenile Court—this transfers parental rights to the local authority. TFTTF

Mental subnormality:

A. is synonymous with intellectual retardation
B. may be defined in terms of a person's social competence rather than his level of intellectual functioning
C. is more likely to have a specific pathological cause when severe than when mild
D. is associated with a higher prevalence of psychiatric disturbance than that in people of normal intellect
E. requires long-term inpatient care in 80% of cases.

According to ICD9 ★, mental retardation refers to 'a condition of arrested or incomplete development of mind which is especially characterised by subnormality of intelligence.' According to standard IQ tests (which have a mean score of 100 and a standard deviation of 15), an IQ below 70 (that is, two standard deviations below the mean) is indicative of mental retardation. This can be further subdivided into mild (IQ 50–70), moderate (IQ 35–49), severe and profound forms. Clinically, it is useful to distinguish people who are mentally retarded with IQs above 50 from those with IQs below this figure (see below).

Unfortunately, the terms mental retardation and mental subnormality have assumed different meanings in different contexts. For example, mental subnormality is defined in the Mental Health Act 1983 in terms of social competence and the capacity to live independently of others, without specific reference to the degree of intellectual impairment. Because of this confusion in terminology, some experts favour the use of the term **intellectual retardation** as a specific clinical term to describe intellectual impairment as measured by IQ testing.

The aetiology of mental retardation is complex and often multifactorial. However, specific aetiological factors include genetic or chromosomal causes (like phenylketonuria and Down's syndrome), abnormalities in the prenatal environment (such as rubella during pregnancy, maternal alcoholism and rhesus incompatibility) and trauma during birth or early infancy (like mechanical injury during birth, hypoxia, status epilepticus and head injury). Such specific aetiological factors are more commonly found in those whose IQ is below 50 than in those with mild mental retardation. In the latter group (which comprises the majority of those with mental retardation), aetiological factors include both parents having low IQs and other influences, mainly environmental. Just how important environmental factors are remains unclear. There is however evidence that social environment may be responsible for a variation in IQ of up to 20 points. Also, mildly retarded people who show no evidence of any of the specific pathological causes mentioned above are almost always from a working-class background.

Mental retardation is associated with a higher than expected incidence of psychiatric disturbance, as well as physical problems such as cerebral palsy, impaired vision or hearing, or epilepsy.

Help and support from professionals and other agencies should be tailored to the individual needs and strengths of each patient and his family, remembering that needs and resources are likely to change over time. A major component in the management of mental retardation is the improved detection and prevention, where possible, of specific factors causing mental retardation.

The majority of mentally retarded people do not require long-term hospital care. Mildly mentally retarded adults are usually able to live in the community and may find employment in sheltered workshops. It is customary now to place even those who are more severely handicapped in the community whenever possible, although a small number of people will continue to require long-term institutional care. FTTTF

Psychiatry and Medicine

MCQ 105

The following statements are true of the term 'psychosomatic':

A. the term 'psychosomatic' refers to a recognised and specific medical discipline

B. psychosomatic medicine is concerned with the relationships between biological, psychological and social factors in disease

C. psychosomatic disorders are always associated with tissue damage or other organic pathology

D. psychosomatic disorders may be considered ones in which psychological factors have a major aetiological role

E. the 'psychosomatic approach' is a specific technique for managing certain types of physical illness

A leading British psychiatrist once wrote that ' "psychosomatic" . . . reflects only a rather muddled phase of specialised ignorance.' The term has been applied in three main areas—the psychosomatic approach, psychosomatic disorders and psychosomatic medicine. Of these, only the last can be defined with acceptable accuracy. Nowadays, the psychosomatic approach is often considered to be synonymous with the holistic approach to medicine, seeing the patient as a total person and not just the carrier of symptoms and signs. However, the use of psychosomatic in this context is confusing and best avoided.

There is no agreement on what constitutes a 'psychosomatic disorder'. For this reason, both the ICD9 ★ and DSM-IIIR ★ classifications have tried to avoid specific reference to this term. According to one definition, psychosomatic disorders are those in which psychological factors give rise to physiological malfunction and associated somatic symptoms in the absence of tissue damage or other organic pathology. However, this definition is somewhat restrictive, since 'physiological malfunction' may itself lead to tissue damage (for example, in the case of stress ulcers). None of the current definitions insists that tissue damage or other organic pathology must be present in all psychosomatic disorders (see also MCQ 108). It is probably best to consider psychosomatic disorders as those presenting with somatic symptoms in which psychological factors play a major aetiological role. However, this is also not entirely satisfactory, because it implies that some diseases are psychosomatic, while others are not. In practice, no such clear distinction is possible. Research has shown the relevance of psychological factors to the aetiology of a wide variety of diseases and it is difficult to separate out those in which such factors are 'of major importance' from others.

Psychosomatic medicine is best defined as the study of the interrelationships between biological, psychological and social factors in maintaining health and in influencing the onset and course of disease. The use of 'psychosomatic' is best confined to this context. In this respect, all medicine may appropriately be viewed as psychosomatic. Although the work done by psychiatrists in some (non-psychiatric) medical settings is sometimes also referred to as psychosomatic medicine, this is more accurately described as liaison psychiatry or general hospital psychiatry.

Some authors have used 'psychosomatic' not only to describe a link between psyche and soma but also to denote the direction of causality, implying that the psychological factors 'cause' somatic consequences (hence also 'somato-psychic'). In this sense, 'psychosomatic' is the same as 'psychogenic'. However, this model is simplistic, ignoring the complexity of the relationship between psyche and soma.

'Psychosomatics' has sometimes been used as the noun derived from 'psychosomatic'. However, in view of the confusion generated by the diverse definitions of the latter, psychosomatics also is a term best avoided. FTFTF

MCQ 106

Stress:

A. may be adequately defined as the physiological response of an organism to an adverse environment

B. is always the result of harmful or pathological change in the interactions between an individual and his environment

C. whatever its form, is best avoided

D. is more likely to affect men than women

E. reactions have consistently been shown to include enhancement of cell-mediated immunity

The term 'stress', like 'depression', is much abused. Stress arises from the interaction of an organism with its environment. Stress may be defined as any change which taxes the adaptation of the individual to his limits, an imbalance between perceived demands on the individual and his perceived capacity. Stress represents the individual's response to stressor(s). Everyday use of the term is confusing because we sometimes refer to stressors as stresses (for example, 'the stresses of modern living'). Although most people associate stress with harmful or adverse change, positive changes are also potentially stressful (for example, a promotion at work). During life, some degree of stress is inevitable. As Hans Selye (attributed with coining the current use of this term in medicine) noted, only death allows complete freedom from stress.

In early studies of stress and its effects, most emphasis was placed on the physiological components of stress. Stress leads predominantly to sympathetic nervous system arousal (the so-called 'fight or flight response') and/or increased activity of the pituitary and adrenal cortex. Although stress was seen in the past as having a final common pathway shared by all individuals (called 'the general adaptation syndrome'), this is now seen as simplistic. Aspects of stress other than the physiological ones have received increasing attention: these include cognitive, behavioural and social aspects, all of which influence an individual's response to a particular stressor. For example, two people may differ markedly in their (cognitive) appraisal of the same stressor, leading to differing responses. The availability of adequate coping strategies as well as social supports is known to moderate the effects of stressors. The predictability of a given stressor, and prior experience of it, are also important. Although there is some evidence that men and women, under defined circumstances, may show differing responses to similar stressors, there is no convincing evidence that men are in general more likely than women to be affected by stress.

The relationship between stress and illness is complex and inadequately understood. Traditionally, stress has been associated as an important aetio-logical factor with a select group of diseases (the 'psychosomatic disorders'—see MCQ 105 and MCQ108). However, it has become clear that the effects of stress are by no means confined to these diseases, but are much more widespread (see MCQ 107).

A variety of physiological changes have been suggested as important in the association between stress and physical illness. For example, some studies have shown raised plasma levels of cortisol and cholesterol associated with particular stressors. It has also been demonstrated that the various components of the immune system can be highly responsive to stress, although the way in which these relate together is as yet poorly understood. A number of research studies have demonstrated impairments in cell-mediated immunity associated with stress, but interpretation of such data is complicated by difficulties in quantifying the stress levels of individual subjects and by the fact that different studies have adopted differing measures of immune function. FFFFF

MCQ 107

The following are statements regarding the relevance of psychosocial factors in physical illness. Which statements are correct?

A. among patients with neurosis, there is a greater than expected risk of death from causes other than suicide or accidents
B. elderly men whose wives have recently died may, as a group, show higher mortality rates from cardiovascular and respiratory causes
C. it has been established that the onset of certain types of cancer is associated with an excess of severe life events
D. in patients presenting with acute appendicitis, an excess of recent life events may be found in those whose appendices turn out to be histologically normal
E. considering the entire adult population of Britain, episodes of illness are randomly distributed

In recent decades, the traditional 'disease' model has been extended to take into account psychological and social factors, whose importance has been demonstrated in a wide variety of physical illnesses (see also MCQ 108).

Not only is psychiatric illness more common among the physically ill than among those in good physical health, but patients with chronic psychiatric problems tend more often than other people to see their general practitioners with physical complaints. As a group, psychiatric patients diagnosed as neurotic have a higher than expected death rate from suicides and accidents, but they also show a significantly increased risk above that expected of death from respiratory, cardiovascular and neurological causes.

Aside from psychiatric illness, other forms of emotional distress can have a profound effect on the onset and course of physical illness. For example, there is some evidence that, among general medical inpatients, emotional distress is associated with a worse prognosis for the physical illness. Among surgical patients, excessive anxiety may lead to increasing analgesic requirements and longer hospitalisations.

The role of stress ★ in physical illness has been of particular interest to researchers in psychosomatic medicine. It was established in the 1930's that episodes of illness are not at all randomly distributed in the population. Some people are more prone to illness than others, and illnesses (both psychiatric and physical) tend to cluster at times of particular stress. Such observations have given rise to numerous studies of life events as antecedents of physical illness. It has been found, for example, that in patients presenting with the signs of acute appendicitis and who come to surgery, those whose appendices are histologically normal show an excess of life events preceding their illness. There is also some evidence that in the weeks before myocardial infarction, male patients will have experienced more life events than other men of the same age and class. In the immediate aftermath of the Athens earthquake of 1981, there was a greater than expected mortality from cardiac causes, particularly among people with underlying coronary artery disease. However, attractive as the idea may be that life events could precipitate many illnesses, the evidence for this (beyond specific research findings like those just mentioned) remains equivocal. For example, one study in the 1960's suggested that some older men were much more likely to die than would be expected in the year following the death of their wives. Subsequent researchers have not all made similar observations. More rigorous research methods, particularly in the measurement of life events, are likely to shed further light on this problem. More attention is now being focused on the possible mechanisms underlying the effects of stress on physical illness (see MCQ 106). TTFTF

MCQ 108

***The following statements are correct regarding the associations between
personality or behaviour, and physical illness:***

A. as a group, people with rheumatoid arthritis have more obsessional person-
   alities than other people
B. characteristic features of Type A behaviour include conspicuous ambition,
   competitiveness and a chronic sense of time urgency
C. an association has been reported between coronary heart disease and the
   Type A behaviour pattern
D. it has been convincingly demonstrated that people who repress their anger
   are less likely than others to develop certain forms of cancer
E. people who worry a great deal are more likely than others to develop
   peptic ulcers

The search for possible causal links between personality and physical illness has
been an important area of research as well as speculation in psychosomatic
medicine.

One psychoanalytic school suggested that certain so-called 'psychosomatic'
illnesses (peptic ulcers were one example) were due to particular psychic
conflicts arising in childhood. Such conflicts, when 'activated' in later life by a
significant life event, gave rise in vulnerable individuals to physiological
changes which in turn produced the physical illness. The psychosomatic
illnesses were all said to be 'conflict-specific', each arising from a different
psychic conflict. Thus in the development of duodenal ulcers, for example, a
life situation that activated conflicted longings for love would be accompanied
(in someone genetically predisposed) by gastric overactivity. Although it remained popular for some decades, this 'specificity' hypothesis lost support
when it could not be confirmed by research.

Numerous research reports have suggested possible associations between
personality traits or types of behaviour and specific illnesses. For example, it
has been suggested that, compared with women who have benign breast
disease, women with breast cancer commonly show longstanding patterns of
extreme suppression of anger and other feelings. Such studies are difficult to
undertake, notably because of the problems involved in quantifying aspects of
personality or behaviour. In any case, causality cannot be inferred from such
associations—it has yet to be shown (for the example above) that chronic
suppression of anger plays a direct role in the aetiology of breast cancer.
Similarly, while worrying excessively may be a feature noted in some patients
who present with peptic ulceration, it has not been established that worry alone
contributes significantly to the aetiology of peptic ulcers.

To date, no component of personality or behaviour has been firmly identified as a major causative factor in any physical disease, with the possible
exception of the 'coronary-prone behaviour pattern'. Features of this include
sustained aggression, ambition, competitiveness and a heightened sense of
time urgency, which together comprise Type A behaviour (Type B being
characterised by the absence of these features). Research has shown that
coronary artery disease is more common among Type A individuals than in
Type B's and there is even evidence that in men who have suffered a

myocardial infarction, behavioural interventions aimed at reducing Type A behaviours decrease the risks of further cardiac morbidity. However, such results will need further replication before the role of Type A behaviour as clarified. The features of Type A behaviour were derived initially from empirical observations of cardiac patients rather than more systematic investigation, and there remains some doubt about the precise meaning of patients' scores on Type A inventories.

While the evidence remains equivocal that certain types of personality or behaviour could give rise to physical illnesses, specific behavioural changes can result from some physical disorders, particularly those involving the central nervous system. For example, frontal lobe damage gives rise to a characteristic behavioural syndrome. The same is said to be true of temporal lobe epilepsy ★, although the evidence for the 'inter-ictal behavioural syndrome of temporal lobe epilepsy' is far from clear. FTTFF

MCQ 109

In a representative British general practice:

A. approximately 5% of consecutive surgery attenders can be recognised as psychiatrically disturbed

B. women are more likely than men to seek help from their general practitioner for emotional problems

C. 40–50% of patients recognised by their general practitioner as psychiatrically ill will be referred to a psychiatrist

D. of those recognised as psychiatrically ill by their general practitioner, a greater percentage of males than females will be referred for psychiatric assessment

E. the only significant predictor of psychiatric referral is the severity of the patient's symptoms

The prevalence of psychiatric morbidity in the community is about 25%. Most of those people who can be recognised in epidemiological studies in the community as psychiatrically ill consult their general practitioner. Up to one-third of general practice attenders will receive a psychiatric diagnosis, although only the minority of these will have presented with predominantly or exclusively emotional or psychological problems. Such complaints are more common among women attending their general practitioner than among men, even allowing for the greater prevalence of psychiatric morbidity in the community among women than men. In other words, even when they can be diagnosed as psychiatrically ill, men are more likely than women to present to their general practitioner with physical complaints.

The general practitioner will himself treat the vast majority (about 95% in a typical British practice) of patients he diagnoses as psychiatrically ill, relatively few being referred for psychiatric assessment. Psychiatric referral rates are slightly higher in the United States, but there the primary health care system differs from that in Britain. Many studies have shown that younger patients are more likely than older ones to be referred for psychiatric assessment. In Britain, male patients are more likely to be referred to a psychiatrist than females. A number of explanations have been suggested to account for this sex difference, including differences between the sexes in the predominant psychiatric diagnoses, the greater pressure of staying off work on the chief breadwinner, usually male, and the fact that males more commonly delay going to their doctor, presenting at a later stage in their psychiatric illness than females and needing different interventions. Referral rates for males and females are not affected by the sex of the general practitioner, although rates may vary from one doctor to the next. However, such possible explanations cannot account for the fact that such a sex difference is absent in psychiatric referrals from primary care physicians in the United States.

The severity of the presenting symptoms is one factor influencing referral, but others are also important, notably the duration of symptoms and their failure to respond to the general practitioner's management. FTFTF

Among patients recognised by their general practitioners as psychiatrically ill:

A. most will be suffering from symptoms of anxiety and/or depression
B. approximately 15% will have a psychotic illness (functional or organic)
C. of every five patients, two will have recovered within one year of the onset of their symptoms
D. of those patients who remain ill one year after the onset of symptoms, more than half will be ill for five years or more
E. those patients diagnosed as clinically depressed usually require treatment with antidepressants

Among patients given a psychiatric diagnosis by their general practitioner, common complaints include anxiety, despondency or sadness, fatigue and insomnia. Half of this patient group will have somatic complaints. Relatively few (approximately 5%) will have a psychotic illness—less than 1% would be expected to have organic psychoses, the remainder having functional psychoses (either schizophrenia or major affective disorder). This contrasts with the diagnostic grouping of psychiatric inpatients, a far greater proportion of whom are psychotic.

The general practitioner's management of this group of patients follows the same principles as for other psychiatric patients, although bearing in mind that their illnesses may not be as severe as those encountered among patients under psychiatric care. The indications for the use of psychotropic drugs are the same in this setting as elsewhere in psychiatry. For example, some cases of depression presenting in general practice show features of melancholia ★, and such cases warrant treatment with antidepressant medication (MCQ 51). Other treatment strategies are more appropriate for other types of depression, which constitute the majority of cases of depression seen in general practice. Reassurance and supportive psychotherapy are important components of treatment. Other types of psychotherapy might be appropriate in individual cases. Social factors commonly play a major role in precipitating and prolonging psychiatric symptoms; such factors should be addressed if possible (for example, a single parent presenting with features of depression may be helped effectively by improving support at home).

In general, psychiatric illness in primary care carries a good prognosis. Of those patients who present as new psychiatric cases, 70–80% will have recovered within one year of the onset of symptoms, and approximately three-quarters will remain symptom-free at three years' follow-up. A minority go on to develop chronic illnesses. Those patients with a poor outcome at one year's follow-up tend to remain ill, over half of this group remaining ill for at least five years. For the majority of patients (those with minor depression or neurotic illnesses) social circumstances (housing, income, social contacts, etc.) are as important as the nature and severity of the symptoms in determining prognosis. TFTTF

MCQ 111

The following statements are true of psychiatric problems among inpatients on a general medical ward:

A. they are almost always associated with a past psychiatric history
B. they occur in approximately one patient in ten
C. they are equally common in male and female patients
D. the most common presenting problems are depression and anxiety
E. the majority of patients concerned are referred for psychiatric assessment

Evidence from research, screening non-psychiatric inpatients, suggests that one-third or more of medical inpatients might warrant a psychiatric diagnosis. The prevalence of psychiatric disturbance is greater in female patients than males, and varies considerably according to specialty. There is, for example, less psychiatric disturbance among surgical inpatients than on general medical wards. Several factors might account for this. Turnover of surgical beds is faster than that of medical beds, thus medical patients have a longer stay in hospital during which psychiatric symptoms might manifest themselves. Another factor is that physicians are more likely than surgeons to admit patients with psychiatric illnesses which present in predominantly somatic form, such as hypochondriasis or the (physical) effects due to alcohol abuse. Although past psychiatric history may help in predicting the likelihood of psychiatric disturbance in medical and surgical inpatients, relatively few of these patients who become psychiatrically disturbed will have a past history of psychiatric illness. In general, their psychiatric disturbance is more short-lived than those of psychiatric inpatients and may carry a better prognosis.

The most common psychiatric problems among general hospital inpatients are depression and anxiety, although in elderly patients, there is a high incidence of organic brain syndromes ★, both acute and chronic. Other problems, like hypochondriasis ★ and hysteria ★, are less common. Some of the psychiatric problems which present in medical settings can be very difficult to fit adequately into the 'conventional' scheme of psychiatric classification (ICD9 ★)—a complete diagnostic formulation might include behavioural, cognitive and psychodynamic factors as well as biological ones.

Despite the high prevalence of psychiatric disturbance, relatively few general hospital inpatients are referred for psychiatric assessment—in Britain, a typical figure would be 2% or less of all admissions to general medical wards. Several factors influence referral to a psychiatrist. Females are referred more frequently than males. Many research studies have reported differences in referral patterns according to age, but no consistent pattern has emerged. Patients with a past psychiatric history tend to attract psychiatric referral more commonly than those without.

There is evidence that non-psychiatric doctors appear not to recognise a proportion of psychiatric disorders as such (an alternative possibility which has not been adequately explored is that doctors do indeed recognise psychiatric problems but are reluctant to acknowledge them because they are less confident about managing them than their patients' physical illnesses). However, it is also true that psychiatric disorders can sometimes be very difficult to recognise in the physically ill. For example, many individual features of depression are commonly found in medical inpatients, and may be due to the physical illness rather than being part of a depressive illness. The severity of the psychiatric disorder appears to be less important than its nature. Thus, for example, a belligerent alcoholic whose behaviour interferes with his medical treatment might be more readily referred than someone who is quite severely depressed. FFFTF

MCQ 112

In medical or surgical inpatients, depression:

A. and anxiety characteristically show a poorer response to treatment in these patients than in psychiatric inpatients

B. is more likely to present diagnostic difficulties in these patients compared with psychiatric inpatients

C. and/or anxiety do not require specific treatments if they represent an understandable reaction by the patient to his illness

D. should not be treated with antidepressants because their side-effects make them particularly hazardous in these patients

E. may present in atypical form

The 'biological' features of depression ★, useful in recognising depressive disorders, occur commonly in physically ill patients who are not depressed. Thus symptoms such as insomnia and loss of appetite are less useful as indicators of depressive disorder in this population than among psychiatric inpatients who are physically well. Conversely, some patients present to their general practitioner or in medical outpatient clinics with somatic symptoms (notably fatigue and lassitude) which turn out to be due to depression. Sometimes, such somatic complaints are accompanied by depressed mood, which offers a useful clue to the diagnosis. In other instances, however, the somatic symptoms predominate the clinical picture, and evidence of depression may be elicited only through thorough and careful clinical assessment. Such as a presentation is known as **masked depression** or **atypical depression** ★.

In this context in particular, an adequate assessment includes not only interviewing the patient but also talking to relatives and others who have known him for some time, and eliciting relevant observations from ward staff. For example, in deciding whether a patient is depressed who has become dysphasic as a result of a cerebrovascular accident (and is thus very difficult to interview), it is helpful to get ward staff to document his pattern of sleeping and eating, how he responds to physiotherapy, to his visitors, and so on.

Even when depression or anxiety appears to represent an understandable reaction to the patient's circumstances, they require comprehensive assessment and appropriate management. For example, anxiety commonly results from a patient's inadequate or incorrect understanding of his illness or its treatment. Helping the patient to understand as much as he feels is necessary to know often leads to an improvement in the patient's mental state. On the other hand, 'blanket' reassurance that he (the patient) should not worry and that he is safe in the hands of the staff may help the staff more than the patient.

Depression is managed in this population as in others, using psychological and biological treatments as indicated. Use of antidepressants depends not on the extent to which the patient's depression is understandable in terms of his circumstances, but on the type of depression.

Antidepressant treatment should be considered when features of melancholia ★ are present (see MCQ 51). Because, in physically ill patients, symptoms such as sleep, appetite and weight disturbance may not be associated with depression, anhedonia ★ may be a particularly important symptom in reaching a diagnosis of melancholia (MCQ 43).

Care must be taken in using antidepressants because their side-effects might prove more hazardous in the physically ill—for example, the potential cardiotoxicity of the tricyclic antidepressants (see MCQ 119) does not usually present a problem in treating someone who is physically fit but may do so if the patient suffers from ischaemic heart disease. In such a case, one of the newer monoamine reuptake inhibitor (MARI) drugs ★ would probably be more suitable.

Depression and anxiety in the physically ill are no less responsive to treatment than in other patients. There is evidence (though largely anecdotal) that episodes of depression of anxiety tend to be much shorter in this group of patients than among those attending psychiatrists. FTFFT

MCQ 113

Which of the following statements are true of pain?

A. pain seldom has a physical origin if its intensity shows marked responses to changes of mood
B. pain thresholds are higher for women than men
C. extroverts tend to complain of pain more than introverts
D. pain due to a recognised organic cause may respond to treatment with tricyclic antidepressants
E. different cultures and ethnic groups may have widely different pain thresholds

The experience of pain is influenced by numerous factors beyond its direct cause. Pain thresholds tend to be lower for women than men; anxiety and fatigue also lower the threshold. Apart from pain thresholds, individuals differ considerably in the extent to which they will complain of pain. Although pain thresholds do not differ across cultures, 'pain behaviour' varies widely from one culture to another. For example, Mediterranean cultures tend to complain more about pain than peoples from Northern Europe. Family attitudes also influence individual responses to pain. Personality is also recognised as important. People who in personality inventories score highly on 'neuroticism' tend to have lower pain thresholds than other people. Extroverts tend to complain more of pain than do introverts.

The individual's response to pain is also affected by the extent to which pain is understood or within his control. Thus preoperative instruction and preparation of surgical patients can lead to decreased requirements for analgesics post-operatively. Patients who are given the chance of regulating their analgesic requirements themselves sometimes require less analgesia than if they have their drug regime regulated by doctors or nurses.

Bearing all these effects in mind, it is hardly surprising that pain which has a clearly organic origin may be responsive to emotional changes, environment and other factors. Thus such responsiveness is an unreliable indication that an individual's pain has little or no organic basis. Pain which is predominantly or wholly psychological in origin tends to have a vague onset and its pattern and symptomatology are often difficult to characterise. However, such pain often starts with some physical cause then persists even when that cause has been adequately treated or removed. Pain is seldom purely 'organic' or purely 'physical'. Careful questioning may lead to evidence of an underlying psychiatric disorder, or at least suggest a psychological or psychodynamic reason to account for the pain. Such pain (with little or no physical basis) tends to respond poorly or in an idiosyncratic manner to conventional analgesics. However, note that the converse is not true—pain which has an organic origin can be ameliorated by some anti-psychotic drugs and by tricyclic antidepressants. Some of the latter appear to have analgesic properties independent of their effects on mood. Other treatments used for pain of psychological origin include relaxation, cognitive therapy ★, behavioural techniques (for example, aimed at reinforcing 'non-pain' behaviour) and exploratory psychotherapy ★.

The DSM-IIIR classification ★ includes the category **psychogenic pain disorder** to describe 'the complaint of pain, in the absence of adequate physical findings and in association with evidence of the aetiological role of psychological factors.' Given the nature and associations of pain, this is a difficult diagnosis to make reliably, and controversy surrounds its use, some authorities arguing that the syndrome of psychogenic pain does not exist as a separate entity. ICD9 ★ contains no diagnostic category equivalent to the psychogenic pain disorder. FFTTT

MCQ 114

Among patients who present with somatic complaints for which no adequate physical basis can be found:

A. they warrant the diagnosis of hypochondriasis in most cases
B. they are always preoccupied with and express concern about their symptoms
C. in most surveys of such patients, females considerably outnumber males
D. depending on the setting in which they present, a substantial minority may turn out to have serious organic illness
E. almost all see their problems in physical rather than psychological terms

Patients who present with somatic complaints for which no adequate physical basis can be found often pose considerable difficulties in diagnosis and management. In most studies of such patients, women considerably outnumber men. While the patients commonly see their problems in entirely physical terms, this is not always true. Some patients whose complaints appear to be entirely physical nevertheless see their problems in psychological (or 'emotional') terms. One factor contributing to this among patients visiting their general practitioners is that some patients see physical complaints as a legitimate reason to consult their doctor, whereas emotional problems may not be. Cultural differences are also very important—the expression of emotional problems in somatic terms is far more common in some cultures than in others.

In any such case, several psychiatric diagnoses must be considered. Somatic complaints are common in depression, and may be the predominant feature (see MCQ 112). In **hypochondriasis** ★, the patient characteristically shows a preoccupation with and concern about some aspect of bodily (or mental) functioning which is considered disproportionate. Some physical disease or abnormality may be present but is considered minor in comparison to the patient's complaints. In other cases, the patient's preoccupation may centre on some 'normal' function. For example, a patient may become very concerned that the pulsation of the superficial temporal artery (often apparent when one lies on one's side) is abnormal. A major problem in making this diagnosis is that the doctor must decide what degree of concern is 'disproportionate'. Such a decision may be quite arbitrary in most cases, apart from those which are extreme. Hypochondriasis is often secondary to some other psychiatric disorder and thorough psychiatric assessment is therefore particularly important.

In **hysterical conversion** ★, the patient may not show concern about the presenting symptoms, even when these are extreme ('la belle indifférence'— see MCQ 67). **Malingering** ★ may have a similar presentation. As with hypochondriasis, hysteria is a difficult diagnosis to make accurately. In one well-known study, 99 patients given a diagnosis of hysteria at one specialist hospital for neurological disorders were followed up. After an average follow up of nine years, 14 were totally disabled and 16 partially disabled due to an organic cause, and 12 had died. This suggests that a substantial proportion of these patients had initially been misdiagnosed as having hysteria. However, other studies have shown that in many cases, the diagnosis of hysteria remains appropriate on following up the patients.

The American DSM-III classification includes the diagnosis of **somatisation**

disorder for patients who present over a period of some years with many different somatic complaints (usually involving many organ systems) for which no physical cause can be found. These symptoms usually start before the patient is 30 years old. Somatisation disorder shares many features in common with Briquet's syndrome ★. Whether either of these conditions exists as a separate syndrome remains controversial. They have no directly equivalent categories in the ICD9 classification.

Other diagnoses are less common but need to be considered. For example, somatic complaints may be delusional, forming part of a psychotic disorder. The delusional nature of the complaints will not always be apparent when the patient presents, but can be elicited by careful history-taking. FFTTF

MCQ 115

The following statements are true of puerperal (post-natal) psychoses:

A. approximately 1 in 200 mothers is affected
B. the onset of symptoms is usually within two days of delivery
C. the onset of psychosis is usually preceded by a period of puerperal depression
D. appropriate treatment may include ECT
E. a history of puerperal psychosis after a previous pregnancy greatly increases the risk of further episodes following subsequent pregnancies

In assessing the mental state of mothers after delivery, it is important to distinguish between 'post-natal blues', puerperal depression and puerperal psychosis.

50% or more of mothers have transient symptoms include lability of mood, tearfulness, anxiety, irritability. They may also complain of poor concentration, although cognition is usually normal on formal testing. The symptoms start a few days after delivery and are transient, resolving spontaneously after a few days without the need for any specific intervention. This clinical picture is known as the **post-natal blues** or **baby blues**. Some researchers have found a higher incidence of the blues among women having their first baby, but the nature and strength of this association remains unclear.

A smaller percentage of mothers (10–20%) develop **post-natal depression**. In addition to the typical symptoms of depression, a mother may become excessively preoccupied with the health of the baby and with her adequacy as a mother. Symptoms usually start three or more weeks after delivery and are commonly associated with practical difficulties involving the baby such as problems in establishing a satisfactory feeding and sleeping routine, sometimes exacerbated by poor support from spouse and family. Not uncommonly, puerperal depression goes unrecognised. Mothers (as well as some of the professionals involved with them) may attribute their symptoms to inadequacy and thus feel guilty about seeking help. This is particularly unfortunate as puerperal depression responds to conventional treatments as do other forms of depression. The condition is associated with a past psychiatric history (particularly depression following previous pregnancies) and is more common than expected in mothers who have experienced the blues shortly after childbirth.

Puerperal psychosis affects approximately 1 in 200 mothers. The psychosis typically has an acute onset, often following one or two sleepless nights. It very seldom starts within the first two days of delivery (when there are usually no manifest mental state abnormalities), but has its onset within the first two weeks. Most cases have pronounced affective symptoms, although some closely resemble schizophrenia. The clinical course sometimes shows marked fluctuations. Treatment follows the same lines as for other psychoses, with emphasis on keeping mother and baby together if possible. If a mother is attempting to breastfeed, problems of drugs reaching the baby via the breast-milk make ECT a particularly useful treatment in some cases. There is often either a family history or past personal history of psychosis. Having had one episode of puerperal psychosis, there is a greatly increased risk of further episodes following subsequent pregnancies (from 1 in 200 to 1 in 7 or even less). TFFTT

174

The following statements apply to the hyperventilation syndrome:

A. most patients with the syndrome will on direct questioning describe symptoms of tetany
B. blood gas estimations commonly reveal a low arterial pCO_2
C. the presence of ECG abnormalities always indicates the need for further investigation of a likely underlying organic cause
D. breathlessness and chest pain, not consistently related to exercise, are common presenting symptoms
E. appropriate treatment includes breathing exercises to discourage patients from diaphragmatic (rather than thoracic) breathing

The term 'hyperventilation syndrome' is usually reserved for overbreathing with respiratory alkalosis in which emotional and/or habit factors play a major aetiological role. It is associated with panic attacks and may present to psychiatrists or general practitioners in this form. It also presents among patients attending medical outpatient clinics. It has been estimated that at least 5% of patients attending cardiology clinics have the syndrome.

Uncommonly, the syndrome will present in acute form with dramatic overbreathing following the subjective sensation of dyspnoea, together with carpopedal spasm, parasthesiae, giddiness and anxiety. The vast majority of cases present with the chronic form of the syndrome, in which the symptoms are not so circumscribed, and may involve any combination of the features of hyperventilation and of anxiety as well as other, more vague, complaints. Breathlessness and chest pain, not consistently related to exertion, are common presentations. In addition to their chronic symptoms, patients will often have acute exacerbations. However, relatively few patients will give a clear history of tetany.

Because of the diffuse presentation of the chronic form of the syndrome, diagnosis depends on maintaining a high index of suspicion for the disorder. Diagnosis is sometimes complicated by the coexistence of the hyperventilation syndrome with cardiac or other organic pathology. The diagnosis can usually be confirmed with a provocation test, in which the patient is encouraged to overbreathe vigorously for 2–3 minutes. If this overbreathing reproduces the symptoms of which the patient complains, this favours the diagnosis. This is the most reliable aid to diagnosis, but there are others. For example, it has been observed that patients who chronically hyperventilate tend to sigh conspicuously during conversation—this has been suggested as a useful clinical sign. Patients who hyperventilate also show a poor ability to hold their breath—unlike people who do not hyperventilate, they are often unable to hold a breath for 30 seconds or longer.

Arterial blood carbon dioxide tension (pCO_2) is low during acute hyperventilation and commonly also in the chronic syndrome, although in the latter, pCO_2 may be within normal limits. After a provocation test, a considerable delay in the return of the pCO_2 to its resting level also supports the diagnosis. Intravenous sodium lactate infusions in some patients mimic the symptoms of their panic attacks, but this is not relevant to hyperventilation. Note that hyperventilation may itself render other investigations abnormal. During hyperventilation, the ECG commonly shows T wave inversion, and EEG abnormalities are enhanced (the routine EEG investigation includes a period of recording during overbreathing for just this reason). Thus the finding of EEG or ECG abnormalities in someone suspected of hyperventilating does not necessarily point to an organic cause as the sole explanation of the symptoms.

Some patients are said to benefit from rebreathing into a paper bag during acute attacks as a way of restoring the pCO_2 to normal levels. However, the treatment of choice is to teach the patient how to breathe appropriately when anxious, particularly training the patient to breathe slowly. Most patients tend to respond to their feelings of dyspnoea with marked thoracic breathing, which exacerbates the symptoms. They are taught to use diaphragmatic breathing instead. In addition to such modifications of breathing, effective treatments also include other anxiety management strategies (see MCQ 61). FTFTF

The following may be appropriate (or expected) emotional responses to being diagnosed as having a terminal illness:

A. denial
B. withdrawal and refusal to speak
C. constantly seeking more detailed information about the illness
D. anger with the doctors
E. depression with marked feelings of worthlessness

People might react to bad news of any sort in a wide variety of ways. There is no single reaction to being told that one has a serious illness which is more 'appropriate' than other reactions. How an individual responds will depend on many factors. These include his understanding of the information he has been given, how prepared he was to receive this information and what strategies he knows which might help him cope with this news. Although responses are ultimately individual, it is often helpful to recognise several phases or components in the responses of patients to bad news (this is analogous to the phase of grief during bereavement ★).

In response to bad news, patients (and relatives) will commonly acknowledge some of the things they have been told but forget or deny others. Denial is a defence mechanism ★ which allows people to come to terms with bad news gradually, at their own pace. Some individuals become very withdrawn and may refuse to talk about their illness. There is some research evidence that denial can, in the short term, have a beneficial effect on the outcome of conditions like breast cancer and myocardial infarction. How denial might operate in these circumstances remains unclear.

The phase of denial is commonly followed by a phase characterised by anger and resentment. 'Why *me*? What have *I* done to deserve this?' are typical responses. Subsequently, there may be a stage of bargaining. For example, a patient might say, '*I* now accept what you tell me about my illness but all I want is to remain well enough to go to my daughter's wedding in September.' Some patients, while not denying their illness, busy themselves in hectic activity in an attempt to avoid thinking about their prognosis. Some patients reach the point where they accept their illness and its outcome, although it is unclear how often this happens.

It must be stressed that, although it may sometimes be useful to recognise these phases when talking with patients and relatives, there is seldom a clear-cut distinction between them in practice. For example, a patient may accept one aspect of his illness while denying another. At any stage during the process of assimilating bad news, a patient might become frankly psychiatrically ill. Depression is the most common response, and should be treated as in other circumstances with antidepressants and/or psychotherapy as appropriate.

Dealing with dying or severely ill patients and their relatives requires patience and sensitivity. The main principle involved is to tailor one's management as a doctor to the needs and strengths of the individual patient and his family. Some will wish to know and understand as much as possible about the illness, others will wish to know less. The doctor must negotiate with each patient what he knows, what he wants to know and how he understands his illness. For the individual patient, all this is likely to change with time and with the course of the illness. It is also important to remember that a patient who asks no questions about his illness is not necessarily showing denial but may be too afraid to discuss it. In this context, doctors have been criticised in the past for participating in a 'conspiracy of silence'. TTTTT

Treatments

Regarding antidepressant drugs:

A. the combination of a monoamine oxidase inhibitor drug and common mild analgesics available without prescription (like aspirin) can produce very severe side-effects

B. newer drugs like mianserin, trazodone and fluvoxamine are particularly useful because they tend to be more efficacious than the tricyclic antidepressants

C. the 'cheese reaction' occurs with some tricyclic antidepressants as well as with the monoamine oxidase inhibitors

D. the acute pharmacological action of the tricyclic antidepressants includes blocking the presynaptic uptake of 5-hydroxytryptamine (serotonin) and/or noradrenaline

E. concurrent administration of a tricyclic antidepressant and a monoamine oxidase inhibitor is absolutely contraindicated because of the risk of serious side-effects

The main classes of antidepressant drugs are the tricyclic antidepressants and monoamine oxidase inhibitors (MAOI). In addition, there are a number of newer antidepressants, some derived from tricyclics (like lofepramine), others having a different structure. There is no evidence that these newer compounds are more effective in treating depression than the older drugs, but they tend to have fewer and less severe side-effects and are thus particularly useful in patients who are especially vulnerable to side-effects, like the elderly or the physically ill.

The tricyclic antidepressants and most of the newer antidepressants can be grouped together as monoamine reuptake inhibitor (MARI) drugs, based on their acute pharmacological effects. Acute administration of a tricyclic antidepressant results in the potentiation of 5-hydroxytryptamine and/or noradrenaline in the brain, by inhibiting their uptake into the presynaptic neurones. The precise relevance of these acute changes to the antidepressant effect of these drugs is unclear. After a few weeks of treatment, receptor changes occur which may be more relevant to the therapeutic action of these drugs. These receptor changes include a decrease in numbers or sensitivity (down-regulation) of beta adrenoreceptors and, in some cases, alpha-2 adrenoreceptors.

The main action of the MAOI drugs is to inhibit the breakdown of monoamines, including 5-hydroxytryptamine and noradrenaline. This also accounts for the '**cheese reaction**', an important side-effect of the MAOIs. Usually, tyramine and other sympathomimetic compounds are broken down by monoamine oxidase soon after ingestion. However, in the presence of MAOI, this does not occur, thus sympathomimetic action is potentiated and severe hypertension may result. For this reason, patients taking MAOI drugs must keep to a diet which avoids high levels of tyramine and similar compounds. Details are usually given to each patient on an 'MAOI card'. Foods to be avoided include meat or yeast extracts (like Bovril, Oxo and Marmite), cheese, pickled herrings and Chianti wine. For the same reason, many proprietary cough mixtures and nasal decongestant drops which contain sympathomimetics must be avoided. However, mild analgesics such as the salicylates do not interact in this way with MAOI drugs. The cheese reaction does not occur with any of the tricyclic antidepressants.

The combination of a MAOI drug and a tricyclic antidepressant can produce very serious adverse effects, including hypertension, hyperpyrexia and fits. It can even prove fatal. However, such effects are most commonly found when one type of drug is discontinued and replaced immediately afterwards by the other, in particular when a tricyclic antidepressant replaces (or is added to) a MAOI drug. A 'washout' period of at least ten days free of medication should be allowed when changing from a tricyclic compound to a MAOI drug, or vice versa. Despite these hazards, it is possible with sufficient care to use the two types of antidepressant concomitantly, and such combined antidepressant treatment is used in 'resistant depression' (depressive illness which fails to respond to an adequate therapeutic trial of one or more antidepressants used alone (see MCQ 52). However, combined treatment with a tricyclic and a MAOI antidepressant should only be started under psychiatric supervision with the patient in hospital. FFFTF

Which of the following statements apply to the side-effects of antidepressant drugs?

A. postural hypotension is one of the common side-effects of phenelzine
B. most tricyclic antidepressants raise the seizure threshold
C. amitriptyline is usually more sedating than protriptyline
D. lofepramine is contraindicated in someone who has recently had a myocardial infarct
E. agranulocytosis is a recognised side-effect of mianserin

Most tricyclic antidepressants produce anticholinergic side-effects such as dry mouth, blurred vision, constipation, urinary retention and sweating. For some patients, they are sufficiently troublesome to persuade the patient to stop treatment. However, the severity of these effects varies from one individual to the next, and there is no convincing way of predicting which patients are likely to suffer severe side-effects.

Anticholinergic effects are less severe and also less frequent with some of the newer MARI drugs, like lofepramine and fluvoxamine.

The tricyclic antidepressants also have a degree of cardiotoxity and should therefore be used with caution in someone with a history of cardiac pathology. Newer drugs like lofepramine, fluvoxamine and mianserin are preferred under such circumstances, being less cardiotoxic. This is one reason why the newer drugs are also safer in overdose, because there is less risk of fatal arrhythmias.

Most tricyclic antidepressants and some of the newer drugs (such as maprotiline and mianserin) should be used with caution in someone with a history of epilepsy or otherwise vulnerable to seizures, because they lower the seizure threshold. However, this is not usually a problem in treating people who are not particularly susceptible to epilepsy, except in overdose, when fits can occur.

Almost all antidepressants are sedating to some extent (the MAOI tranylcypromine is unusual in that it has a stimulant effect, and protriptyline and viloxazine are also said to be stimulant). However, some are more sedating than others. This is important clinically as someone with severe insomnia might benefit from a sedating antidepressant given as a single dose at night, while sedation might be undesirable for another patient with a retarded depression. Sedative antidepressants include amitriptyline, mianserin and trazodone, while those which are less sedative include imipramine, clomipramine, lofepramine and fluvoxamine. However, this only serves as a very rough rule of thumb because in practice, there are considerable differences between patients in the extent to which they are sedated by any drug.

In addition to these common side-effects, individual drugs have important side-effects of which the prescriber must be aware. For example, a few cases have been reported of agranulocytosis associated with mianserin and a regular review of the full blood picture is thus essential when mianserin is prescribed.

Postural hypotension is a common side-effect of all MAOI drugs, including phenelzine, and may even occur at therapeutic doses. In addition, dizziness and headaches may occur. The main hazard in using MAOI drugs is the 'cheese reaction' ★. TFTFT

Regarding treatment with lithium:

A. dysarthria and ataxia are likely to occur when plasma levels are above 2.0 mmol/l
B. nephrogenic diabetes insipidus due to lithium therapy may be successfully treated using a thiazide diuretic
C. this may give rise to weight gain
D. diarrhoea is a side-effect
E. concomitant administration of diazepam is contraindicated

The side-effects of treatment with lithium can be divided into those which occur early in treatment (within days), intermediate-term effects and long-term effects.

Early side-effects may include nausea, disturbances of bowel function (constipation or diarrhoea), weight gain, thirst and dry mouth. These effects are usually transient and require no specific treatment. After longer use, effects which may occur at therapeutic doses include tremor, thyroid disorders (either hypothyroidism or, less commonly, hyperthyroidism) and nephrogenic diabetes insipidus. These symptoms may respond to lowering the dose of lithium and are reversible with discontinuation of lithium. The tremor sometimes responds to propranolol. Nephrogenic diabetes insipidus sometimes responds to careful treatment with thiazide diuretics—this combination can be hazardous (see MCQ 54) and such treatment requires careful monitoring and usually also lowering the dose of lithium. The main late complication of therapy with lithium, which occurs after prolonged administration of high doses of lithium (to give serum levels of 1.3–1.5 mmol/l), is chronic renal failure.

Symptoms of lithium toxicity (which occurs at serum levels of 2.0 mmol/l and above) include nausea, ataxia, dysarthria, coarse tremor and impairment of consciousness.

Besides the effects of combining lithium and sodium-losing diuretics like frusemide and the thiazides, lithium potentiates muscle relaxants and there is also some evidence that, in combination with persistently high doses of haloperidol, toxic effects may be produced on the brain. Lithium produces no significant interaction with diazepam. Other aspects of treatment with lithium are considered in MCQ 54. TTTTF

MCQ 121

Which of the following statements regarding the benzodiazepines are correct?

A. short-acting benzodiazepines (like lorazepam) represent the best available treatment for panic attacks
B. their use may lead to an increase in irritability and aggressive behaviour
C. rebound insomnia may occur on discontinuing a benzodiazepine hypnotic taken regularly for 1–2 weeks
D. longer-acting benzodiazepines produce milder but more prolonged withdrawal reactions than shorter-acting compounds
E. tolerance to some of the effects of the benzodiazepines may occur after only 2–3 doses of the drug

Recognition that the benzodiazepines may rapidly give rise to dependence has limited their use as hypnotics and anxiolytics.

Dependence ★ occurs in 15–20% of long-term users of benzodiazepines and one study has estimated that one-third of those taking a benzodiazepine for six months or more develop dependence. Withdrawal symptoms are often similar to those the drug was initially prescribed to treat, such as rebound insomnia and anxiety. Other psychological symptoms include perceptual disturbances (such as heightened sensitivity to sensory stimuli), phobic symptoms, depression, derealisation and depersonalisation, and irritability. Acute psychotic episodes may occasionally occur. A wide variety of somatic symptoms also occur, including nausea, diarrhoea, palpitations and parasthesiae. Rapid withdrawal leads to an increased risk of epileptic seizures.

Dependence may develop very rapidly. Rebound insomnia may be evident after only 1–2 weeks' continuous use of a benzodiazepine hypnotic. In general, the more gradual the rate of withdrawal, the less severe the withdrawal syndrome. Longer-acting benzodiazepines (such as flurazepam) tend to produce a milder but more prolonged withdrawal syndrome than short-acting preparations (like triazolam and lorazepam).

Tolerance may develop very rapidly to some of the effects of the benzodiazepines after 2–3 doses. Tolerance develops more rapidly to the hypnotic effects of the benzodiazepines than to their anxiolytic effects. However, there is evidence that they are no longer effective as anxiolytics after 1–4 months' continuous use.

Apart from dependence, long-term use of the benzodiazepines may give rise to other problems. These include episodes of depression and a chronic apathetic state described as 'emotional anaesthesia'. They may also have a disinhibitant effect, which may sometimes give rise paradoxically to outbursts of aggression or to antisocial acts such as shoplifting or sexual offences.

Because of such problems, prescription of benzodiazepines as hypnotics or anxiolytics is best limited to brief courses (less than two weeks) at the lowest dosage and, where possible, intermittently rather than continuously. Other treatments may be more appropriate than the benzodiazepines in managing insomnia or anxiety—for example, relaxation training and other techniques of behaviour therapy ★. A benzodiazepine should only exceptionally be used as sole treatment for anxiety or insomnia. FTTTT

Regarding antipsychotic drugs:

A. haloperidol is more sedating than chlorpromazine
B. thioridazine is virtually free of anticholinergic effects
C. the phenothiazines are sometimes used as adjuncts in weight reduction
D. galactorrhoea is a side-effect of phenothiazines
E. pigmentary retinopathy is a recognised complication of use of thioridazine at doses about 800 mg daily

Most antipsychotic drugs in common use are phenothiazines or butyrophenones. The phenothiazines can be further divided on the basis of their chemical structure into aliphatic compounds (such as chlorpromazine), piperidines (such as thioridazine) and piperazines (like trifluoperazine). Of the butyrophenones, haloperidol is the most commonly used in psychiatry. Haloperidol resembles the piperazines more closely than the other types of phenothiazines. Pharmacologically, the phenothiazines and most other antipsychotic drugs act as dopamine antagonists.

The antipsychotic drugs all share a range of side-effects, including extrapyramidal effects ★, sedation and antiadrenergic and anticholinergic effects. The extrapyramidal effects include acute dystonias ★, akathisia ★ and parkinsonism ★. The aliphatic phenothiazines are the most sedative of the three groups, and the piperidines have most anticholinergic action. Thus haloperidol has less sedative effect than chlorpromazine and thioridazine has most anticholinergic effect. As anticholinergic drugs are used to treat the extrapyramidal side-effects of the antipsychotic drugs, it follows that thioridazine and other piperidines are less likely than the other groups of drugs to produce extrapyramidal symptoms. However, thioridazine also has considerable antiadrenergic effects, which contribute to the postural hypotension some patients experience on this drug. The anticholinergic effects of thioridazine may also cause confusion in the elderly.

Other side-effects of the antipsychotic drugs include galactorrhoea and menstrual disturbances which may be associated with elevated levels of prolactin and also weight gain (the mechanism of which is uncertain). In addition, there are important side-effects associated with individual antipsychotic drugs. Doses of thioridazine exceeding 800 mg daily can cause an irreversible pigmentary retinopathy. Chlorpromazine may cause cholestatic jaundice as an idiosyncratic reaction. FFFTT

MCQ 123

Which of the following apply to long-term treatment with antipsychotic drugs?

A. using depot (injectable) antipsychotic drugs overcomes the 'first-pass' effect which occurs with oral preparations
B. plasma prolactin levels usually return to normal in the first 6–9 months of antipsychotic treatment
C. 'drug holidays' effectively reduce the risk of developing tardive dyskinesia
D. long-term treatment with antipsychotic drugs is more effective in treating the negative symptoms of schizophrenia than the positive ones
E. tolerance to their effects is common

The main rationale for the long-term administration of antipsychotic drugs in schizophrenia is the prevention of relapse. Although effective in suppressing the positive symptoms ★ of schizophrenia, maintenance medication has no direct demonstrable effect on the negative symptoms.

The most consistent endocrine response to administration of antipsychotic drugs is elevation of plasma prolactin (see MCQ 122). With continuing drug treatment, the prolactin levels usually remain elevated, although they may gradually fall towards normal levels in a few individuals.

Tardive dyskinesia ★ is a chronic movement disorder due to the antipsychotic drugs. There is no evidence that prescribing antipsychotic drugs in separate courses with 'drug holidays' between each course reduces the incidence of tardive dyskinesia. Low dose and intermittent drug treatment strategies are currently being explored, but their therapeutic value has yet to be fully established.

Depot antipsychotic drugs are no more efficacious than oral preparations, but can be useful when patients are unable or unwilling to take their oral antipsychotic medication regularly. The two types of drug differ in their bioavailability. Oral preparations are to some extent converted to inactive metabolites by non-specific enzymes in the gut wall and are also rapidly metabolised during 'first-pass' through the liver. These problems are avoided by using depot preparations. There is no evidence that significant tolerance develops to the pharmacological actions of the antipsychotic drugs. TFFFF

Regarding the extrapyramidal side-effects of the antipsychotic drugs:

A. drug-induced dystonia may develop acutely 24 hours or longer after a single dose of a dopamine antagonist
B. acute dystonic reactions are more likely to affect elderly patients than others
C. akathisia is invariably a transient phenomenon lasting a few days
D. drug-induced parkinsonism is characterised by low frequency resting tremor rather than muscle rigidity
E. acute dystonic reactions show more favourable responses than akathisia to anticholinergic drugs

Acute dystonic reactions are abnormal postures produced by sustained muscle spasms. They have a reported incidence in patients on antipsychotic medication of 2–10%. Children and young adults are the most commonly affected. The reactions usually occur within 24–48 hours of starting antipsychotic treatment (90% occur within four days of starting antipsychotic medication) but may occur on withdrawal of antipsychotic medication.

The muscles of the head and neck are usually affected. Symptoms may include trismus, blepharospasm, facial grimacing, oculogyric crises, dysarthria, dysphagia, glossopharyngeal contractions, spasmodic torticollis and retrocollis. These muscle spasms are often painful and frightening, although subtler forms, such as tightness of the shoulder and neck muscles or difficulty in speaking and chewing may hardly be noticed by the patient and may only be discovered by direct questioning.

Acute dystonic reactions can be effectively relieved within minutes by intravenous or intramuscular anticholinergic drugs.

Akathisia affects 20% of acute psychiatric patients given antipsychotic drugs. Patients feel unable to remain still, and feel a compulsion to move which may be particularly referable to the legs. Many patients complain that the condition is least tolerable when they are required to stand still. In addition, characteristic restless movements may be observed, including rocking from foot to foot or treading on the spot when standing, and shuffling or tramping of the legs and repeated leg-crossing, or swinging of one leg when sitting. Patients with severe akathisia are unable to tolerate any position, sitting, lying or standing, for more than a few minutes.

Although acute akathisia may improve with dose reduction, it tends to persist, often with a fluctuating course over many years. The only reliable treatment for akathisia is withdrawal of antipsychotic medication, a strategy which may be hazardous for some psychiatric patients. Anticholinergic drugs have an uncertain reputation as a specific drug treatment. Some investigators claim success with these agents while others report that the response is unsatisfactory. Recent work suggests that modest doses of beta-adrenoreceptor blockers like propranolol can produce a rapid and marked improvement.

Drug-induced parkinsonism has an estimated incidence of 10–15% in patients on antipsychotic drugs. Although its course is inadequately understood, it has been suggested that this condition is commonest in the first three months of treatment with antipsychotic drugs and subsequently tends to improve spontaneously. The condition shares many signs and symptoms with idiopathic Parkinson's disease, but is more likely to present with muscular rigidity than with a festinant gait or with the characteristic resting 3–5 Hz 'pill-rolling' tremor of Parkinson's disease, although other types of tremor are commonly seen. Patients with drug-induced parkinsonism often show persistent resistance to passive movements of the limbs (**'lead-pipe' rigidity**) or a succession of resistances which are rapidly overcome, known as **'cogwheel' rigidity**. Disturbance of postural reflexes can lead to complaints of unsteadiness, a festinant (or hurrying) gait and falls. The gabellar tap sign often fails to habituate—patients continue to blink in response to a regular, rapid tap between the eyebrows. Other symptoms, such as bradykinesia with lessening of spontaneity, a 'mask-like' impassive face, paucity of gesture and slow, monotonous speech, may be mistaken for retarded depression (so-called akinetic depression—see depressive stupor ★). Anticholinergic drugs such as procyclidine and orphenadrine are generally beneficial in treating drug induced parkinsonism (see also MCQ 127). TFFFT

Tardive dyskinesia:

A. is thought to involve supersensitivity of dopamine receptors in the nigro-striatal system
B. usually shows some improvement on treatment with anticholinergic drugs
C. may be improved by increasing the dose of the antipsychotic drug
D. its development is strongly dependent of the dose of antipsychotic medication and the duration of its administration
E. is more common in schizophrenic patients with a history of positive symptoms than in those without

Tardive dyskinesia is usually a later side-effect of antipsychotic drugs than akathisia and parkinsonism. It comprises involuntary movements predominantly affecting the mouth, tongue and face, but may also include the trunk and extremities. Advancing age is the only variable consistently associated with increased prevalence and severity of tardive dyskinesia. However, there is accumulating evidence that the prevalence of tardive dyskinesia is increased in schizophrenic patients with predominantly negative symptoms ★.

Tardive dyskinesia is thought to be due to hypersensitivity (increased receptor numbers) of postsynaptic dopamine receptors in the nigrostriatal region of the basal ganglia. Withdrawal of the antipsychotic drug tends to give an acute exacerbation of the condition rather than an improvement, while raising the dose of the antipsychotic drug usually produces temporary alleviation. Treatment with anticholinergic drugs invariably exacerbates tardive dyskinesia, although there is no good evidence that chronic prescribing of anticholinergic medication increases the risk of the condition developing. TFTFF

MCQ 126

Which of the following are recognised features of the neuroleptic malignant syndrome?

A. muscular rigidity
B. sudden pyrexia
C. low serum creatinine phosphokinase
D. a strong association with haloperidol administration
E. dantrolene has been reported as an effective treatment in some cases

The neuroleptic malignant syndrome is a serious but rare complication of treatment with antipsychotic drugs. The syndrome comprises: muscular rigidity, with cogwheeling as in parkinsonism or less commonly the waxy flexibility of catatonia; diffuse and coarse tremor; fluctuating levels of consciousness or the akinetic mutism of stupor; a sudden pyrexia often with profuse sweating; and tachycardia and a labile blood pressure. Laboratory tests reveal a leucocytosis and a marked elevation of serum levels of muscle enzymes like creatinine phosphokinase.

The aetiology of the syndrome is unknown, apart from the fact that it represents an idiosyncratic response to antipsychotic drug administration, not dependent on the dose of the drug or the duration of its prescription. No particular antipsychotic drug or class of drugs has been clearly implicated as being more likely to produce the syndrome than others.

Management consists of immediately stopping the antipsychotic drug treatment and admitting the patient to an acute medical bed. Dantrolene may ameliorate the rigidity and hyperthermia in some cases. Dopamine agonists such as amantadine, bromocriptine and L-dopa have also been reported as beneficial. Intravenous lorazepam has been used to combat the catatonic features. Complications of the syndrome include pneumonia, pulmonary embolism and dehydration leading to acute renal failure. The mortality has been estimated as 20%. TTFFT

Anticholinergic drugs:

A. can be drugs of abuse
B. can interfere with the absorption in the gut of antipsychotic drugs
C. should be prescribed to all schizophrenics at the start of treatment with antipsychotic medication as prophylaxis against the development of extra-pyramidal side-effects
D. commonly produce a measurable improvement in cognitive functioning in chronic schizophrenic patients
E. can produce toxic confusional states in the elderly

Following the introduction of antipsychotic drugs in Britain in the 1950's, it became widespread clinical practice to prescribe anticholinergic drugs routine-ly at the onset of treatment, to prevent the development of extrapyramidal symptoms. The evidence against such prophylactic prescribing is first, that anticholinergic drugs exacerbate tardive dyskinesia ★. Secondly, the preva-lence of extrapyramidal symptoms decreases with time, and withdrawal of anticholinergic agents after three months leads to a relapse of extrapyra-midal symptoms in only a small proportion of patients (approximately 10%). Thirdly, the administration of anticholinergic drugs is associated with undesir-able side-effects such as agitation, anxiety, tremor, blurred vision, confusional states, precipitation of glaucoma, urinary retention and toxic psychosis (acute brain syndrome ★). These side-effects are most likely to occur in elderly patients. In addition, anticholinergic drugs may interfere with the therapeutic action of concurrently prescribed antipsychotic drugs, both by reducing their absorption from the gut and possibly by antagonising their effects in the central nervous system. Also, there is limited evidence that anticholinergic drugs may be responsible for cognitive impairment in schizophrenic patients, producing defects in memory, attention and concentration.

In view of these findings, it is now generally recommended that anticho-linergic agents should not be routinely prescribed, and when indicated for the management of extrapyramidal symptoms, they should be prescribed for limited periods only. However, patients are often reluctant to reduce or discontinue their anticholinergic drugs.

There is increasing evidence that anticholinergic drugs exert central effects on psychological functions such as mood, arousal, aggression, sexual behaviour, biorhythms and sleep. They can sometimes produce mania-like states. Perhaps as a consequence of these effects, there are reports of anticholinergic agents being used as drugs of abuse. TTFFT

MCQ 128

Regarding electroconvulsive treatment (ECT):

A. it can be effective treatment for catatonic stupor
B. administration of ECT lowers the blood pressure
C. it involves the administration of a muscle relaxant before the fit is induced
D. unilateral ECT stimulating the non-dominant hemisphere cause less post-ictal confusion and memory disturbance than bilateral ECT
E. before it can be administered, two psychiatrists must agree that it is necessary in every case

The main indication of ECT is in the treatment of depressive illness with particular features (see MCQ 53). However, it may also be beneficial in certain cases of acute schizophrenia, for example those presenting with catatonic stupor. It is commonly used in the post-partum psychoses not only because it is often rapidly effective but because of the hazards to the infant in giving psychotropic drugs to a mother who is breastfeeding (see MCQ 115).

Raised intracranial pressure is considered an absolute contraindication. Unless the treatment is considered a life-saving measure, it should be avoided if the patient has had a myocardial infarction in the previous six weeks. Blood pressure rises during ECT, thus patients with severe hypertension, a history of cerebral haemorrhage or with cerebral or aortic aneurysms are also at greater risk than other patients. As with all treatments, likely benefits of the treatment must be balanced against the possible risks of the treatment as well as those involved in allowing the disorder to continue.

In ECT, a seizure is induced by an electric current to the head. The patient is given a short-acting anaesthetic drug, a muscle relaxant and an anticholinergic agent, together with oxygenation. As a result, the seizure is 'modified' and does not produce a generalised convulsion, being manifest only as a brief movement of facial muscles. Because of the administration of anaesthesia, patients should be fasted for a minimum of six hours before the treatment.

Short-term side-effects of ECT include headache, confusion, memory disturbance, nausea and vomiting, and parasthesiae. All these effects are transient. Whether ECT produces long-term memory impairment remains uncertain although currently available evidence indicates that if this occurs, it is a very subtle effect which tends not to show up on standard tests of memory. Unilateral ECT stimulating the non-dominant hemisphere is associated with less confusion and memory disturbance in the immediate post-treatment period when compared with bilateral ECT.

As with other treatments requiring an anaesthetic, written consent is required for ECT. If the patient agrees to the treatment, this can be given without further consultation, even when the patient is detained in hospital under the Mental Health Act. If the patient is unwilling or unable to give consent, it is common practice to place the patient on Section 3 of the Mental Health Act. Under Section 58 of the Mental Health Act, the opinion of an independent psychiatrist, appointed by the Mental Health Act Commission, must then be sought before the treatment can be administered. However, like other treatments, under common law, ECT may be commenced without obtaining consent (either from the patient or a Mental Health Act Commission doctor) when it is urgently necessary as a life-saving measure. TFTTF

Which of the following statements about psychotherapy are true?

A. transference is a process by which a patient displaces onto his therapist feelings, attitudes and ideas derived from important figures in his (the patient's) past
B. transference reactions occur in behavioural psychotherapy
C. countertransference is a process by which the patient displaces his feelings onto a third party, not involved in the therapy
D. having few or no defences is an indication of emotional maturity
E. the unconscious refers to all mental processes of which the person is not aware

Transference is a process by which one person displaces feelings, attitudes or ideas derived from people who were significant in his past onto another person. This is likely to occur whenever two people meet and is not a process exclusive to any particular type of psychotherapy. However, it is particularly important in psychoanalysis and other types of exploratory (dynamic) psychotherapy in which transference forms one of the major 'tools' of the therapy. Transference reactions lead the patient to invest in his therapist characteristics, attitudes and feelings which may be totally inappropriate. In some types of exploratory psychotherapy, this process is encouraged by the therapist remaining as 'anonymous' as possible, for example by giving very little of his own personality into the therapy sessions and by sitting out of direct view of the patient. By **interpretation** and other techniques, transference reactions may be changed or modified during therapy, allowing the patient to establish a more realistic appraisal of people with whom he comes into contact.

The equivalent process in the therapist to the patient's transference is **countertransference**. Feelings and attitudes from the therapist's past may cloud his sensitivity and understanding of the patient's emotions. Thus, for example, a young doctor may find himself responding to some people of his parents' age as though they had the same feelings and attitudes as his parents. Clearly, this complicates and may hinder the therapeutic relationship, which is one reason why it is the standard practice in some types of psychotherapy (like psychoanalysis) for the therapist to receive supervision of his own personal therapy. In a broader sense, countertransference includes the feelings which the therapist experiences that originate with the patient. Although they may not be recognised or described as such, countertransference feelings occur universally in medicine but may be particularly striking in managing some patients such as certain individuals who are terminally ill. For example, nursing and medical staff may feel very angry towards a patient, much of the anger originating with the patient himself but not necessarily expressed openly.

According to psychoanalytic theory, we all have primitive emotions and drives which, were they within our awareness, would arouse great anxiety because they conflict with consciously-held ideals and socially acceptable norms. We use **defence mechanisms** to keep these primitive urges beyond consciousness—they remain unconscious. The **unconscious** refers to mental contents and processes kept away from conscious awareness by repression and other defence mechanisms. Mental processes whose exclusion from consciousness does not rely on defence mechanisms do not strictly form part of the unconscious. This may apply, for example, to some of the automatic thoughts which are important in cognitive therapy ★.

Defence mechanisms are universal and important in preserving our emotional integrity—it is when our defence mechanisms break down that symptoms ensue. A variety of different defences have been described, including denial, displacement (in which hostile feelings which cannot be expressed towards an authority figure, for example, are taken out on someone less powerful), repression (keeping the unacceptable urges in the unconscious) and sublimation (in which the anxieties is dissipated by channelling energy into positive acts or ways of life such as creativity). TTFFF

Psychotherapy in general:

A. always requires special training
B. very seldom requires the therapist to be directive (as opposed to interpreting and reflecting feelings and observations back to the patient)
C. almost always involves patient and therapist concentrating on discrete problems which have been defined at the start of therapy
D. may cause the patient to become dependent on the therapist
E. may exacerbate a patient's psychiatric disorder rather than improving the symptoms

Psychotherapy may be defined as the treatment of mental and emotional disorders based primarily on verbal and nonverbal communication with the patient. This definition embraces a wide variety of different therapies, from those which require lengthy training (such as psychoanalysis) to supportive psychotherapy, which is practised daily by all those working with the mentally or physically ill.

The psychotherapies can be distinguished according to their theoretical or empirical bases, although they share the fact that each aims to offer the patient a way of understanding his disorder. Psychoanalysis, for example, is based on ideas derived from the work of Freud and his followers that certain types of emotional disturbance reflect the conflicts between feelings and attitudes which are conscious and others which are beyond consciousness (see MCQ 129). Cognitive therapy ★ has a different theoretical basis. The fact that different types of psychotherapy do not share a common basis does not mean that they are mutually exclusive or incompatible—some problems may be better understood in terms of one model, other problems (even affecting the same patient) in terms of another model.

The psychotherapies also differ in the ways they are applied in practice. Thus psychoanalysis and other types of long-term exploratory psychotherapy involve patient and therapist meeting regularly, sometimes over a period of several years. The therapy does not focus on discrete symptoms but aims to give the patient a better understanding of important unconscious mechanisms which cause conflicts within him. The therapist is not directive—the patient is not told what to do or offered advice. By contrast, behaviour therapy requires the therapist to be directive and involves a time-limited course of treatment agreed at the start by therapist and patient (see MCQ 133).

Like other forms of treatment, the psychotherapies may have hazards in individual cases. For example, the patient may become over-dependent on the therapist, particularly in those forms of therapy in which the 'contract' between patient and therapist is loosely defined. Some psychotherapies, such as different types of exploratory psychotherapy, can be very stressful to the patient. In the case of someone with a history of schizophrenia or affective illness, for example, exploratory psychotherapy may exacerbate symptoms or even precipitate an episode of acute illness. FFFTT

Which of the following apply to supportive psychotherapy but not to exploratory psychotherapy?

A. transference reactions are irrelevant
B. the patient's defences are reinforced rather than confronted
C. the emphasis is on the patient's present rather than his past
D. unconscious mechanisms are emphasised
E. minimal use is made of interpretation

Exploratory psychotherapy (also known as (psycho)dynamic or interpretive psychotherapy) aims to allow the patient to gain insight into unconscious mechanisms which give rise to painful emotions. Transference ★ reactions are encouraged and interpreted where appropriate, allowing the patient to make links between his present feelings and attitudes and those from the past. For example, a man is very troubled by the fact that he is easily angered by the attitudes of his superiors at work. He is liable to become angry with the therapist whenever the therapist declines to offer him advice or more frequent therapy sessions. The therapist observes to the patient that whenever he (the therapist) is perceived as an authority figure, the patient's reaction appears to be similar to that at work. The therapy allows the patient to trace this back to his feelings towards his father—he wanted his father to be a powerful and protecting figure as well as someone he could look up to. However, he had always perceived his father as none of these things, but rather as a weak and ineffectual person. This allowed him to gain insight into his behaviour towards authority figures—he tended to 'test them out' in various ways to see if they would prove as weak as his father had been. Note that **insight** ★ in this context means something different from that which is lost in the psychoses—none of us should ever expect to gain complete insight (in the psychodynamic sense) into our feelings and attitudes.

Supportive psychotherapy, by contrast, aims to optimise the patient's present and future level of functioning rather than to help him gain insight into how his emotional conflicts originated. Thus minimal use is made of interpretation. Transference reactions are not encouraged (as they are in exploratory psychotherapy) but they do occur (as in any other type of psychotherapy) and must be acknowledged and dealt with. One example would be the patient become excessively dependent on the therapist, seeing him as a substitute for parents or spouse.

In exploratory psychotherapy, the patient's defences are examined and sometimes confronted as part of the process of gaining insight. In supportive psychotherapy, the opposite is the case—the patient's defences are reinforced as far as possible. FTTFT

Which of the following suggest that a person is likely to be unsuitable for exploratory psychotherapy?

A. the patient is unable to see his problem in psychological terms
B. low intelligence and/or poor verbal fluency
C. being unable to make a regular commitment to therapy over a period of at least 18 months
D. the patient is totally unable to remember any of his dreams
E. the patient has been diagnosed as schizophrenic and currently has delusional beliefs

In assessing a patient's suitability for exploratory psychotherapy, several criteria are useful. The patient must have the motivation to pursue psychotherapy, to wish to gain insight and to change, and must also see his problems in psychological terms. Someone who has hysterical paralysis may wish to regain normal limb function but may be unable to see his problem in psychological terms. Although the interpretation of dreams is an important component of some exploratory psychotherapies (Freud referred to dreams as 'the royal road to the unconscious'), being able to remember one's dreams is not essential for therapy.

The patient must also be able to form and sustain a relationship with the therapist—whether or not this is likely may be evident from other relationships in the patient's life. Someone who has led a chaotic and nomadic lifestyle and has never had any close relationships may be unable to form a therapeutic relationship. The patient should also have sufficient 'inner strength' to cope with the emotional conflicts aroused by the therapy. Thus a person who copes with crises by taking repeated overdoses is unlikely to prove suitable for exploratory psychotherapy. Being able to express one's thoughts and feelings is clearly an asset in psychotherapy, but patients of quite limited intelligence can undergo therapy provided that the therapist acknowledges and works within the patient's limitations.

Because exploratory psychotherapy is likely to be stressful, it may precipitate an episode of psychiatric illness in a patient who is particularly susceptible to this, like someone with a history of schizophrenia or of mania. For this reason, many psychotherapists do not accept such patients into therapy, and being actively psychotic would in most cases exclude exploratory psychotherapy. Some psychotherapists go even further in insisting that during their therapy, patients should take no psychotropic medications.

Although exploratory psychotherapy often continues over a period of years, this is not essential and does not apply to **brief focal psychotherapy**. Here, although the therapy follows psychodynamic principles, it is focused on specific problems and limited to frequent sessions over a period of usually six to nine months. TFFFT

MCQ 133

Behavioural psychotherapy (behaviour therapy):

A. is indicated for problems which have discrete symptoms which are observable, either directly or indirectly
B. is the treatment of choice in the management of compulsions in obsessive compulsive disorder
C. does not directly address the underlying causes of the problem being worked on
D. uses the techniques of systematic desensitisation and flooding
E. usually depends for its success on the patient being on little or no regular medication

In exploratory psychotherapy, the patient's 'symptoms' (defence mechanisms, transference reactions, and so on) are usually inferred from the therapy—they are usually not directly observable and cannot be quantified. By contrast, the use of behaviour therapy depends on being able to define the patient's problem(s) in terms of phenomena which can be observed and quantified. For example, compulsive rituals can be directly observed, the circumstances under which they are performed documented, and the amount of time spent performing them measured. Similarly, with an agoraphobic patient, the main symptom can be defined and quantified—someone who is still able to make short trips alone is less severely affected than a person who is completely unable to leave the house. In some instances, the symptom can only be observed indirectly, as in the case of obsessional ruminations—here, reliance is placed on the patient's report of the ruminations. Similarly, an anxious patient can be taught to quantify his anxiety on a 0–10 or 0–100 scale.

It follows from this that the problems amenable to behaviour therapy are those which can be defined and quantified in behavioural terms. These include phobias, compulsions, certain types of sexual problems and tension headache, amongst others. In addition, behavioural techniques are useful in managing inappropriate behaviours in those with chronic psychiatric illness or mental subnormality (such as self-injurious behaviour in the mentally handicapped).

A behavioural treatment begins with a thorough **behavioural analysis**, the definition and properties of 'target behaviour(s)' or other symptoms which will form the focus of the treatment. For each target symptom, information is gathered not only about the behaviour itself but also about antecedents (such as cues which might spark the symptom off) and consequences of the behaviour (such as the amount of time during the day used up in carrying out compulsive rituals and the consequent restrictions on everyday activities). An important part of therapy is getting the patient to keep adequate records of these factors.

In addition to the need to define and quantify the target symptoms, therapy depends on the symptoms being repetitive and sufficiently frequent to allow modification. If there is no recognisable pattern to the behaviour, behavioural interventions are very unlikely to help. Similarly, if the symptoms of which a person complains only occur twice a year, it is difficult to design a workable behavioural programme. Behavioural treatment programmes are time-limited, the number of sessions of treatment agreed with the patient at the start of treatment as part of a comprehensive therapeutic 'contract'.

The treatment is focused on the symptom(s) themselves and is not directly concerned about how the symptoms originally started. This 'here-and-now' approach contrasts with that in exploratory psychotherapy. In treating someone with a spider phobia, for example, the focus in exploratory psychotherapy would be in discovering how this problem could be understood in terms of the patient's past and also the symbolism of the spider (what spiders represent for that individual). In behaviour therapy, these questions are not directly addressed.

Systematic desensitisation ★ is a common technique in behaviour therapy, applied when anxiety is a feature of the patient's problem. Patient and therapist together devise a hierarchy of anxiety-provoking stimuli and the patient is exposed to the stimuli in order, starting with the least threatening. Thus someone with a severe spider phobia might start by looking at a picture of a spider and, once able to do this without excessive anxiety, progress to turning the pages of a book on animals in which photographs of spiders occur, then observing a small plastic spider, and so on. Relaxation techniques are sometimes helpful adjuncts to this process. **Flooding** involves exposing the patient to the most severe feared stimulus at the start. Various operant conditioning techniques are also used, based originally on work with laboratory animals by Skinner and others. These techniques include **positive reinforcement** (giving some form of reward after appropriate behaviour) and **aversion** (giving a noxious stimulus to eliminate unwanted behaviours). **Modelling** of appropriate behaviours by the therapist is a useful component of many treatment programmes.

The success of behaviour therapy does not depend on whether or not the patient is taking any psychotropic medications. However, this may be important in some circumstances. For example, reduction of anxiety by exposure to anxiety-provoking stimuli is less successful if the patient takes excessive quantities of alcohol or tranquillisers.

Because behaviour therapy does not address the underlying causes of particular behaviours, it might be assumed that, having removed one symptom, another might arise in its place—so-called **symptom substitution**. In practice, this occurs only rarely. Why this is has yet to be adequately explained. TTTTF

MCQ 134

Cognitive therapy:

A. is a form of psychoanalysis
B. is a specific technique which aims to improve memory and other intellectual functions
C. may be helpful in the treatment of patients whose delusions respond poorly to antipsychotic drugs
D. is based on the theory that cognitions or 'automatic thoughts' may be taken as valid even when they are abnormal or wrong
E. is a useful treatment for some neurotic conditions

The term 'cognition' can be confusing, as it is used in different contexts with slightly different meanings. In the mental state examination, cognitive impairment means an impairment of higher intellectual functions. However, 'cognitions' also describe a person's thoughts and the ways they are dealt with by the mind—the term covers beliefs, interpretations, expectations and other aspects of thinking. Cognitions form a link between the individual's emotional responses to perceptions or experiences and the actual perceptions themselves. We use (and need) cognitions to interpret our immediate experiences. Although cognitions occur within the conscious mind, people are usually unaware of them—they happen automatically, hence they are sometimes described as **automatic thoughts**. Everyone develops a particular cognitive style, which is like an individual repertoire of automatic thoughts and ways of dealing with them. The same experience or perception may evoke quite different emotional responses in different people, depending on their cognitions. For example, one person might get very angry when someone tries to jump a queue in front of him, while another person hardly notices the same incident at all. Despite such individual differences, cognitions are normally taken for granted and regarded as implicitly true.

Cognitive theory suggests that some psychiatric disorders, notably neuroses and some cases of depression, are linked to abnormal cognitions. Indeed, some theorists go further, arguing that abnormal cognitions are the direct cause of some psychiatric conditions. For example, a man who has a social phobia may, every time he enters a novel social situation, get the automatic thought that he will appear socially inept, make a fool of himself and thus be a laughing stock. Not being aware of these automatic thoughts, all he experiences is intolerable anxiety. This leads him to avoid such situations, which serves to set up a vicious circle.

Cognitive therapy aims to make the individual more aware of his or her automatic thoughts, allowing them to be examined and, where appropriate, changed. Thus at the start of treatment, the social phobic might agree to keep a record of social situations he finds difficult, together with the thoughts that such situations generate. There are particular techniques which can be used to 'capture' automatic thoughts in this way. Patient and therapist then collaborate in assessing how valid the thoughts are and, where appropriate, finding arguments against them. For example, the social phobic might be encouraged to remember social situations in which he has been successful and also to examine whether a minor social slip will inevitably lead to complete disgrace, as his original thoughts implied. This process is termed **cognitive restructuring**. With practice, the patient can become aware of the automatic thoughts as they occur and can deal with them before becoming excessively anxious.

Clearly, cognitive therapy is likely to be useful in those psychiatric disorders which can be understood in terms of abnormal cognitions and which are amenable to collaborative work by patient and therapist. Thus this form of therapy is not used in the treatment of the psychoses. Although delusions may bear some superficial resemblance to automatic thoughts, these two phenomena are different, most notably because by definition, delusions, being held with unshakeable conviction despite contrary evidence, are not amenable to the kind of examination and cognitive restructuring described above.

Unlike psychoanalysis and other forms of exploratory psychotherapy, cognitive therapy does not require the existence of an unconscious. Cognitions are already 'known' to the patient, or directly accessible, unlike unconscious mechanisms, which can only be reached via psychoanalytic techniques like the use of the transference ★. Another difference between exploratory psychotherapy and cognitive therapy is that the latter (like behaviour therapy ★) is structured and involves a number of specific techniques (like those used to elicit automatic thoughts). This makes it easier to research the efficacy of cognitive therapy compared with exploratory psychotherapy. A treatment plan using cognitive therapy often involves behavioural components (like getting the social phobic to expose himself to social situations). However, unlike behaviour therapy, cognitive therapy does not focus attention primarily on symptoms but rather on the cognitions that underly these. FFFTT

MCQ 135

Which of the following criteria have to be met in order to detain a patient in hospital under the Mental Health Act 1983 (other than on an 'emergency' section)?

A. there must be a risk to the health or safety of the patient and/or other people
B. the patient must in every case have a mental disorder
C. a psychiatric assessment must have been made by an experienced psychiatrist
D. the patient's nearest relative, as defined by the Mental Health Act, must make the application for admission
E. a social worker must witness the fact that the patient refuses voluntary admission

Section 2 of the Mental Health Act 1983 relates to the compulsory admission of patients to hospital. There must be an application for admission and two medical recommendations. The application can be made either by the patient's nearest relative (the Act defines who constitutes the nearest relative) or by an 'approved' social worker (a social worker recognised by the local authority as having experience in mental health assessment). In practice, it is usually preferable for a social worker to make the application for admission rather than involving the family too directly at a time which is often very stressful for everyone concerned. The two doctors making the medical recommendations, like the social worker who makes the application for admission, must both have personally interviewed the patient. At least one of the doctors must, according to the Act, 'have special experience in the diagnosis or treatment of mental disorder', and one or both the doctors should preferably have known the patient before the time of this assessment. In practice, the two doctors involved are usually the patient's general practitioner and an experienced psychiatrist (usually a senior registrar or consultant).

In order to recommend the patient's compulsory admission to hospital, the doctors involved must satisfy themselves that the patient is suffering from a mental disorder (further details are included in the Act itself) of sufficient severity to warrant hospitalisation, and that this is necessary 'in the interests of his own health or safety or with a view to the protection of other persons'. Clearly, it is not necessary to use the Mental Health Act if the patient agrees to come into hospital voluntarily. This is one point which the doctors and social workers would wish to pursue with the patient. The Act requires the 'approved' social worker to satisfy himself the compulsory detention of the patient is the best way of providing care and medical attention for the patient. However, those cases in which the application for admission is made by the nearest relative will not necessarily involve a social worker.

Section 2 allows the detention of a patient for psychiatric assessment for up to 28 days. Under **Section 3**, the patient may be kept in hospital for **treatment** for up to six months. Like Section 2, Section 3 requires an application and two medical recommendations. The criteria for use of Section 3 are similar to those of Section 2, but the nature of the psychiatric disorder must be defined in more detail (it is assumed that 'assessment' has been undertaken and the patient's disorder may thus be assigned a diagnosis).

Section 4 is for emergency admissions for assessment, and permits the detention of the patient in hospital for up to 72 hours. Criteria for its use are the same as for Section 2 but only one medical recommendation is required (not necessarily by an experienced psychiatrist). It is used when admission is urgently necessary and the time required to get a second medical recommendation would involve undesirable delay. TTTFF

MCQ 136

Which of the following statements are true of the Mental Health Act 1983?

A. the Mental Health Act permits any patient already admitted to hospital to be detained in hospital on the authority of the consultant in charge of his care for up to 72 hours for a mental health assessment

B. a patient who has acute appendicitis but refuses consent for laparotomy may be treated without his consent under Section 3 of the Mental Health Act

C. anyone may be removed from his home to a hospital or other 'place of safety' by a policeman who suspects that that person may be mentally ill

D. general practitioners may make medical recommendations for the compulsory admission to hospital of patients for psychiatric assessment

E. social workers who are 'approved' as defined under the Act are empowered to remove anyone with a psychiatric disorder from his home and bring him to hospital

A policeman may, under **Section 136** of the Act, remove anyone whom he suspects may be mentally ill from a **public place** (but *not* a private home) to what is defined in the Act as 'a place of safety' (usually the nearest hospital), where the patient can be detained for up to 72 hours, to allow his assessment by a psychiatrist and an approved social worker.

A person may not be removed from his home to hospital, either by a policeman, or by an 'approved' social worker alone. The social worker can make an application for compulsory admission, but there has in addition to be at least one medical recommendation before the patient can be brought to hospital (see MCQ 135).

Section 5(2) is another 'emergency' section, permitting a patient who is already an inpatient (not necessarily in a psychiatric unit) to be detained in hospital for up to 72 hours by the consultant in charge of his care (or the 'nominated deputy' of that consultant) if the doctor believes that detention of the patient under Section 2 or Section 3 might be appropriate (MCQ 135). This allows the patient to be kept in hospital until a formal mental health assessment is possible.

Note that the 'emergency' sections—Sections 4, 5(2) and 136—all permit the patient to be kept in hospital for up to 72 hours. In all cases, the aim is to allow more thorough assessment of the patient. A general practitioner may recommend a patient's compulsory admission to hospital under Section 4 (MCQ 135).

The Mental Health Act is concerned only with the assessment and treatment of psychiatric disorders and has no relevance to the case of a patient who refuses laparotomy for appendicitis. Whether and when one intervenes under such circumstances is a complex question addressed (at least in principle) by the common law. TFFTF

Clinical Cases

Clinical Case 1

Patient 1

Arthur R, a 40-year-old executive with a large motor company, has recently separated from his wife. Mr R attends his general practitioner's morning surgery complaining of poor concentration and a decrease in his work performance. The history further reveals two weeks of initial insomnia but Mr R denies any sadness. At this point, the general practitioner should:

A. prescribe a tricyclic antidepressant as Mr R is likely to be depressed following the breakup of his marriage
B. prescribe a short course of benzodiazepine hypnotic to help him sleep
C. contact his wife to arrange marital therapy
D. ask him to come back later for a full social and psychiatric history
E. prescribe a multivitamin preparation as a 'tonic'

As is often the case when a patient first contacts his general practitioner, Mr R denies any strong emotions. He admits to difficulty sleeping, poor concentration and reduction in his capacity to work. Although these are all features of depression, Mr R denies any sadness or anxiety. A further clue suggesting depression as a likely diagnosis is his recent separation from his wife. About 80% of cases of depression seen in general practice arise out of adverse social circumstances or recent life events.

It would be premature to prescribe an antidepressant until there has been opportunity to establish the diagnosis better. Similarly, it is too soon to assume that separation from his wife is a major cause of his problem (it might have resulted from his difficulties rather than contributing to their cause). Faced with such problems, patients sometimes request a 'tonic' from the doctor, but at this stage, this is clearly little more than a placebo and should not be prescribed. However, symptomatic treatment for his insomnia is appropriate as fatigue might be exacerbating his difficulties at work. Ideally, a full history should be obtained from the patient when he first presents. However, often this is not possible during a busy surgery, even when the general practitioner is familiar with the patient's background. It would be appropriate to prescribe a short course of a short-acting benzodiazepine hypnotic, such as temazepam.

The most important next step is to get a full history from the patient and also, if possible, from someone else, such as his wife or a colleague from work or both. Approaching another informant requires the patient's agreement. FTFTF

The general practitioner decides to prescribe amitriptyline 25 mg at night as an antidepressant and gives Mr R an appointment to return in two weeks. Mr R does not attend this appointment, but returns one month later and is obviously worse. He tells the doctor that he finds mornings particularly difficult to cope with. He has been off work for a week and requires a certificate. He tells the doctor that he stopped taking the tablets after two nights because they gave him a dry mouth.

This time, the doctor asks Mr R to return for a longer appointment after the regular surgery. On enquiring further, the general practitioner is surprised to learn that Mr R left his wife and two children, rather than the other way round. Mr R agrees to allow the doctor to speak to his wife, who still lives with the children in the family home while Mr R himself rents a flat nearby.

Mrs R turns out to be very worried about her husband. She felt that he had become increasingly morose and introspective for several months before leaving home. She thought that he had a mistress but was surprised to learn from a friend that he was alone in his new flat. Mrs R had been quite relieved in a way to get him out of the house, because he had been upsetting the children (aged 8 and 10). She had initially expected him to return home when he got fed up of living alone, but was gradually losing hope of this happening. Until a few months ago, their marriage had been a happy one and Mrs R could think of no reason why he was behaving in this way other than attributing his problems to the 'male menopause'. It had not occurred to her that he might be ill.

At this stage, possible diagnoses include:

A. the male menopause
B. a mid-life crisis
C. endogenous depression
D. alcoholism

The male menopause may or may not exist, but is in any case of no help in planning the further management of Mr R's difficulties. A mid-life crisis carries the implication that Mr R is going through a phase of questioning aspects of his life such as his work and his marriage, finding them unsatisfactory, and making a last attempt to change them before middle and old age creep up on him. Forty is rather young for this, but it is nevertheless a possibility. However, it is more important at this stage to exclude depression as a diagnosis. Factors favouring endogenous depression (melancholia) are his lack of concentration and his own report of feeling worse in the mornings than at other times. The lack of any clear precipitant to his disturbance also points to the diagnosis of melancholia—although most episodes of depression (whatever the type) have recognisable precipitants, absence of such a precipitant is associated more often with melancholia than with other types of depression. However, the type of sleep disturbance expected in melancholia is terminal rather than initial insomnia. Alcoholism must be considered as a possibility in a middle-aged male executive who is behaving out of character and who has a mood disorder. FTTT

The general practitioner decides to refer Mr R to the psychiatric outpatient clinic at the local hospital, with a diagnosis of '? endogenous depression'. While waiting for the appointment, Mr R takes an overdose of amitriptyline, which he has stored since discontinuing his course of treatment. Fortunately, he is discovered quite accidentally by a neighbour and admitted urgently to hospital.

Clinical Case 1

The following symptoms and signs of overdose might be anticipated:

A. hepatic necrosis
B. profound unconsciousness
C. cardiac arrest
D. pinpoint pupils
E. epileptiform seizures

Lowering of consciousness is likely, and may be profound. Tricyclic antidepressants in overdose may also result in epileptiform seizures or cardiac arrest. Hepatic necrosis occurs with paracetamol overdose but not with the tricyclic antidepressants. However, multiple drug overdose should always be suspected where there is evidence of serious suicidal intent, as is possible in this case (he had saved his medications and was discovered only by accident). Where appropriate, initial management of patients admitted after drug overdose should include screening for other drugs likely to have been taken, such as paracetamol and salicylates. The anticholinergic effects of amitriptyline would cause mydriasis rather than constriction of the pupils. FTTFT

On transfer to the psychiatric ward, Mr R admits that he is disappointed that he is still alive. He is agitated and unable to eat or sleep. Physical examination shows obvious weight loss but no other abnormal physical signs.

His wife visits and is very upset seeing him as he is. He admits to her that he left home because he felt completely worthless but had not felt able to tell her this before.

At a further interview, Mr and Mrs R agree that their marriage has been a good one, but Mr R insists that he is unworthy of it, especially as he knows that he has been performing so badly at work that he would inevitably lose his job and was expecting a letter of dismissal any day. Enquiries at his place of work gave a rather different picture. Although the people at work had been aware of his recent difficulties, he is regarded as a valued executive who, when well, applies himself well and enthusiastically to his work.

Mr R denies excessive drinking, and his wife confirms that he has not been abusing alcohol. However, Mr R's father drank to excess and his mother had had episodes of severe depression, requiring repeated hospital admissions in the latter part of her life for electroconvulsive treatment and other treatments. She died in a mental hospital.

Mr R readily acknowledges that he needs treatment and is willing to receive this in hospital.

On the basis of the information so far available, Mr R is likely to be suffering from:

A. alcoholism
B. alcohol dependence
C. melancholia
D. some other type of depression
E. personality disorder

His belief that he is utterly worthless is not borne out by the observations of his wife or his work colleagues—this belief is probably delusional. This, together with the positive family history of depression, support the features already noted favouring melancholia as the diagnosis. The information available gives no grounds to diagnose alcoholism, alcohol dependence or personality disorder. FFTFF

What action would it be appropriate to consider taking now?

A. prescribe amitriptyline 150 mg at night
B. start a course of ECT after obtaining the patient's consent
C. see Mr and Mrs R together to discuss their marriage in more detail to show Mr R that he is not a failure
D. prescribe chlorpromazine 200 mg daily to treat his delusions of worthlessness
E. prescribe a monoamine oxidase inhibitor because he previously had side-effects from amitriptyline
F. place Mr R under Section 3 of the Mental Health Act because he is potentially a danger to himself in view of his previous suicide attempt

The diagnosis of melancholia predicts a positive response to physical treatments such as tricyclic antidepressants or ECT. Most psychiatrists would not consider using a monoamine oxidase inhibitor drug as the first-line treatment of melancholia. The presence of delusions of worthlessness make this a psychotic depression. At this stage, discussions with his wife are unlikely to help and may increase Mr R's agitation. Psychotic depression often fails to respond adequately to antidepressants alone, and usually requires the addition of an antipsychotic drug such as chlorpromazine (this alone would not lift the depression). Explanation and encouragement are likely to help Mr R tolerate the side-effects of a tricyclic antidepressant, but one of the newer monoamine reuptake inhibitor antidepressants could be considered as an alternative to amitriptyline. All antidepressants require two weeks' administration before their effects on depression are likely to become apparent—ECT is often more rapidly effective, and is particularly advantageous in the presence of delusions. If Mr R were not prepared to remain in hospital to have treatment, his depression and the considerable risk of further suicide attempts would make it appropriate to consider placing him on Section 3 of the Mental Health Act (a 'treatment' order would be appropriate rather than an 'observation' order—Section 2—as the diagnosis is sufficiently clear that a particular treatment approach is indicated). However, Mr R is willing to remain in hospital to receive treatment, thus compulsory detention under the Mental Health Act is not indicated. TTFTFF

Mr R consents to have ECT. After his second ECT treatment, Mr R is showing signs of improvement and following ten treatments (3 per week), he is well enough to go home. He is discharged home on a maintenance dose of a tricyclic antidepressant (for example, amitriptyline 100 mg at night).

Clinical Case 2

Patient 2

A late middle-aged man is brought into casualty at 10.00 p.m. by the police under Section 136 of the Mental Health Act, having been found wandering in his pyjamas in the rain one hour earlier. The police report that he appeared confused and incoherent and was seen to be making the sign of the cross repeatedly when apprehended. When examined in casualty, he cannot give a coherent history and is disorientated in time and place. He is able to give his name and address and is not known to the police. Examination reveals a well-nourished man dressed in expensive pyjamas. He is clean but dishevelled and slightly dehydrated, with a tachycardia and raised pulse pressure. He appears fearful and is sweating and complaining of spiders crawling over his skin. He accuses the casualty officer of stealing his spectacles. There is no evidence of any significant physical illness, in particular no focal neurological signs or abnormalities in the cardiovascular system. He is sedated with chlorpromazine 100 mg i.m. because of his disturbed behaviour and admitted to the psychiatric ward for investigation and treatment.

Immediate management should include:

A. thorough physical examination
B. administration of further sedative drugs
C. blood sugar and urine examination
D. regular observation of vital functions and fluid balance
E. urine specimen for drug screen

The first priority is to identify any treatable causes for his condition, while monitoring vital signs and fluid intake and output. A thorough physical examination should be carried out paying particular attention to the neurological system and to any signs of infection or cardiovascular disease. Blood sugar should be measured to exclude hypoglycaemia and urine analysis carried out to exclude diabetes or renal pathology. Metabolic disorders should be excluded by measuring plasma urea and electrolytes, liver function tests, calcium and phosphate and if thyrotoxicosis is suspected, plasma thyroxine. Further sedation should be avoided if possible until the situation is clearer. A urine specimen for drug screen will reveal the presence of benzodiazepines, amphetamine-like drugs, opiates or cannabis. TFTTT

The following history is obtained from previous medical notes and from his sister. He is 59 years old, and from a well-to-do family. There is no family history of psychiatric illnesses. Since his divorce 12 years ago, he had been living with his elderly and infirm mother, who died ten months ago. Although he had been an intelligent man with a degree in architecture, he had never obtained satisfactory employment and had had a drink problem for the last ten years. He has been hospitalised twice (7 and 8 years ago) for a behavioural disturbance associated with alcohol abuse and had a history of ingestion of 'TCP' mouthwash. There had been no recent history of alcohol abuse but large numbers of empty bottles of 'TCP' mouthwash and benzodiazepine hypnotics were found in his flat. He had recently led a 'Walter Mitty' existence with exaggerated ideas about his wealth and importance. He has a tendency to squander his money and is irresponsible about his financial affairs, engaging in unrealistic and unprofitable business deals.

The differential diagnosis includes:

A. delirium tremens
B. Wernicke's encephalopathy
C. acute brain syndrome (acute confusional state) due to another cause
D. mania

The differential diagnosis is that of an acute brain syndrome (acute confusional state). The commonest cause in this type of patient is delirium tremens, and he presents some of the classic features of this disorder, namely confusion, autonomic arousal and visual and tactile hallucinations. There is a history of alcohol abuse, and benzodiazepine withdrawal would also predispose to this condition. 'TCP' mouthwash contains phenol, salicylic acid, chloride and bromide and could have contributed to the toxic state. Wernicke's encephalopathy should also be considered even though he does not show the classic triad of confusion, nystagmus and ophthalmoplegia, since a high incidence of pathological changes characteristic of this disorder have been found at post-mortem, even when the condition was not suspected during life. Other causes of acute brain syndromes also need to be excluded. Mania is less likely, but should be considered because of the history of grandiose ideas and financial irresponsibility. TTTT

Further management should include:

A. administration of sedative drugs
B. treatment with thiamine and other B group vitamins
C. an intramuscular injection of Modecate 50 mg
D. ECG and chest X-ray

Once delirium tremens is suspected, treatment with sedative drugs is mandatory, although care must be taken not to sedate the patient too heavily. Large doses of thiamine and other B group vitamins should be given to prevent permanent neurological sequelae, particularly Korsakoff's psychosis. Antipsychotic drugs should be avoided if possible, since they lower the epileptic threshold. TTFT

The patient is started on chlormethiazole ('Heminevrin' caps ii q.d.s), thiamine 100 mg q.d.s. and 'Parenterovite' 2 ml i.m. daily. Because of continuing disturbed behaviour, he is also prescribed chlorpromazine 100 mg t.d.s. as required. He is started on a fluid chart and his vital functions are monitored. 24 hours after admission, he has a series of grand mal seizures which respond to diazepam 20 mg i.v. Physical examination again reveals no focal neurological signs.

Clinical Case 2

At this stage:

A. chlorpromazine should be stopped
B. the dose of chlormethiazole should be increased
C. treatment with phenytoin should be started
D. an urgent CAT brain scan should be arranged

It is likely that this patient has suffered withdrawal seizures, and chlorpromazine, which lowers the epileptic threshold, should be discontinued. Chlormethiazole should be increased if liver function is not impaired. This is itself an anticonvulsant, and further anticonvulsant treatment at this stage is unnecessary. There is no evidence of focal neurological damage and a CAT brain scan can be carried out when the acute condition has improved. TTFF

Chlorpromazine is discontinued. The patient has no further seizures and over the next few days becomes more lucid. He takes fluids and food satisfactorily. Urine output is normal as are his ECG and chest X-ray. Biochemistry reveals a slightly raised alkaline phosphatase and aspartate transaminase, but the gamma-glutamyl transpeptidase is normal and the ESR is 3. Urine drug screen reveals the presence of benzodiazepines. Chlormethiazole is reduced and stopped after ten days. Thereafter he is fully orientated but at times irritable and disinhibited, making advances towards female staff. He is unconcerned about his dress and hygiene and easily loses his way around the ward, although he is quite active and, at times, proves difficult to restrain from leaving the ward. Cognitive testing reveals an amnesic period surrounding the time of admission to hospital with patchy recent and long-term memory. There is some confabulation. He shows slight nominal dysphasia and poor visuospatial function.
Likely diagnoses now include:

A. alcoholic dementia
B. Korsakoff's psychosis
C. manic illness
D. Alzheimer's disease

The differential diagnosis is now that of generalised cerebral dysfunction with evidence of dysfunction in the frontal lobes (disinhibition, irritability, lack of concern over dress and hygiene), parietal lobes (poor visuospatial function, losing his way around the ward), and possibly temporal lobes (memory disturbance). With the history of alcohol abuse, alcoholic dementia is likely. Other causes of dementia are much less likely but should be considered. He is rather young to have Alzheimer-type senile dementia (SDAT), and Alzheimer's disease itself (a form of pre-senile dementia) is uncommon. Also against SDAT is the negative family history.

His presentation is consistent with Korsakoff's psychosis, but this is unlikely because memory disturbance is not the most prominent feature in his presentation and also because he appears overactive (apathy is more common in Korsakoff's psychosis). TFFF

Further investigation should now include:

A. EEG
B. CAT brain scan
C. cerebral arteriography
D. psychometric testing

Investigations should now be carried out to exclude treatable causes of dementia and to confirm the diagnosis. An EEG may confirm organic brain damage and should also be carried out in view of the previous seizures. A CAT brain scan will reveal gross cerebral damage and exclude treatable focal pathology. Formal psychometric testing will be of use in the assessment of current mental functioning and assist in rehabilitation. TTFT

EEG reveals generalised slow waves, but no epileptic activity. Moderate asymetric dilation of the lateral ventricles and mild cerebral atrophy is shown on the CAT scan. Psychometry reveals a verbal IQ of 120 and a performance IQ of 100. There is a large subtest scatter suggesting an organic pathology. Memory testing is consistent with an organic deficit.

Because of continuing disinhibition and behavioural disturbance, chlorpromazine 100 mg t.d.s. is restarted. Over the next few weeks behaviour improves with no further seizures or confusional episodes. There is a slight improvement in memory but he remains cognitively impaired. He takes more care of personal hygiene and dress but is unable to perform easily simple tasks at occupational therapy and requires supervision and encouragement to carry out day-to-day tasks on the ward.

Rehabilitation should include:

A. sheltered housing
B. sheltered employment
C. abstinence from alcohol
D. lithium carbonate
E. transfer to part III accommodation

The patient clearly requires day-to-day supervision, and some form of sheltered accommodation would be desirable. Hopefully sheltered employment could be arranged in the future, while day centre attendance would be useful in the short term. Alcohol consumption is absolutely contraindicated and a careful check should be made of any drug ingestion or self-medication. He is most likely to benefit from a medium- or long-stay hostel or group home environment. TTTFF

Accommodation is arranged at home, pending longer-term arrangements. Local social services are asked to visit him at home to monitor how he is coping, and the family agree to provide more support than before his admission. His sister makes an application for the Court of Protection to appoint a Receiver to handle his considerable finances, and this is awarded by the Court after receiving medical and social reports. He is discharged to the outpatients on chlorpromazine 100 mg t.d.s. (this is subsequently reduced and finally discontinued). Six months later he remains abstinent and has obtained employment as a voluntary helper in a school. Repeat cognitive testing reveals no improvement in his IQ and residual cognitive deficits of a similar order to those prior to discharge.

The final diagnosis is:

A. alcoholic dementia with delirium tremens
B. Alzheimer's disease
C. bipolar affective disorder

The picture was complicated by his abuse of benzodiazepines and 'TCP' mouthwash. TFF

The most likely outcome if he abstains is:

A. complete recovery
B. slow deterioration
C. rapid dementia
D. swing into a depressive phase

The natural history of alcoholic dementia is stability or even improvement with abstinence in the short term. The long-term prognosis is uncertain. FFFF

Patient 3

Errol K, a 21-year-old West Indian man, is brought to the casualty department by his brother, who reports that the patient has been acting strangely for the last few weeks. He has stopped attending his engineering course at the local technical college and has spent most of his time locked in his bedroom. He has often been heard shouting unintelligibly and tends to stay awake most of the night. When approached by members of the family he has been uncommunicative, suspicious in his attitude and occasionally aggressive, although he recognises them as always.

The patient is virtually mute, and appears agitated, fearful and distractable. He continually glances at a particular area on a blank wall in a way that suggests he is experiencing visual hallucinations.

The differential diagnosis at this time includes:

A. mania
B. alcoholic hallucinations
C. temporal lobe epilepsy
D. drug-induced psychosis
E. encephalitis

The symptoms described are compatible with all the diagnoses listed except temporal lobe epilepsy. Although visual hallucinations do occur in temporal lobe epilepsy, the length of time of the disturbance and the lack of impairment of consciousness render it an unlikely diagnosis. However, there are rare cases of patients with temporal lobe tumours developing a psychiatric illness resembling schizophrenia. Encephalitis is a possible diagnosis but not the most likely. The level of consciousness would be expected to fluctuate and there are commonly neurological signs such as ocular palsies, nystagmus, ataxia and upgoing plantar responses. The story that he tended to stay awake most of the night, together with the observations in casualty suggesting that he may be psychotic, raises the possibility of mania. However, this is unlikely because, far from being grandiose and expansive, he has been uncommunicative at home, locking himself in his room, and is now virtually mute. Alcoholic hallucinosis is rare. Thus, of the diagnoses listed, a drug-induced psychosis is the most likely at this stage. FTFTT

Brief physical examination is essentially normal. The patient does not smell of alcohol and the family confirm that there is no reason to suspect alcohol abuse. The patient is admitted to hospital immediately.

The following investigations are indicated as soon as possible:

A. thorough physical examination
B. thyroid function tests
C. serological tests for syphilis
D. urine screen for drugs
E. CAT brain scan
F. psychometric assessment

Clinical Case 3

The urine screen for drugs and the complete physical examination are required immediately. The tests for syphilis and of thyroid function should be carried out as soon as possible. Where the facilities exist, it is advisable to have a CAT brain scan carried out in a young person experiencing the first serious psychotic episode in order to exclude a cerebral tumour and to provide a baseline scan against which later scans could be compared. However, this procedure requires the cooperation of the patient and may be delayed until his mental state is more settled, unless there is a particular reason to suspect a tumour (for example, focal neurological signs). Psychometric assessment also requires the patient's full cooperation. The results of psychometric assessment would not alter his management at this stage and psychometry is therefore not indicated. TTTTFF

All investigations prove to be normal except for the urine analysis which reveals cannabis.

On admission he is observed for two days free of medication. He becomes slightly calmer and more communicative with nursing and medical staff, telling them that he has been chosen by God to carry out a special mission. God knows his thoughts and speaks to him, puts thoughts into his head, and sometimes takes control of his thoughts and actions in a way that he describes is like a robot that has been programmed by a computer. In addition, the newscasters on the television are sending him coded messages which are designed to confuse him and prevent him carrying out his mission.

Following this description the patient appears to exhibit the following symptoms:

A. first-rank symptoms of schizophrenia
B. ideas of reference
C. thought blocking
D. ideas of passivity
E. tactile hallucinations

His mental state reveals thought insertion, a Schneiderian first-rank symptom. The experience that God is taking control of his thoughts and 'programming' them is a passivity phenomenon, which is also a first-rank symptom. He apparently also has auditory hallucinations, but not all such hallucinations are first-rank symptoms. He has a delusional belief that he has been chosen to carry out a special mission—this may be a primary delusion (also a first-rank symptom) or it could be secondary to his hallucinations. TTFTF

He is given a provisional diagnosis of schizophrenia. Although a cannabis-induced psychosis remains a possible diagnosis in this man, such episodes are usually short-lived, and in addition to hallucinations and delusions, patients usually show emotional lability and disorientation, neither of which has been marked in this case. Treatment is begun with oral chlorpromazine and the patient steadily improves over the next two weeks. He adopts a normal sleep pattern and becomes more rational and relevant in his talk. However, he has a number of specific complaints. Which of these are likely to be attributable to his antipsychotic medication?

A. a seriously sunburned face
B. a feeling of restlessness
C. tinnitus
D. tingling in his fingers
E. inability to obtain an erection

Tinnitus and parasthesiae are the only complaints which are unlikely to be due to his medication. Restlessness is probably due to akathisia. Some patients on chlorpromazine develop a photosensitive rash. Sexual dysfunction is not uncommon. TTFFT

After four weeks, the psychotic symptoms have reduced in intensity, but the patient has become lethargic with flattened affect, spending most of the day sitting around on the ward. He spends weekends at home with his family. He returns from one weekend leave more agitated and deluded but settles over a day or so back on the ward. The family say that he has been demanding to return home but they do not yet feel he is well enough to be discharged. This has apparently led to heated arguments at home. The patient's mother visits him almost every day on the ward for an hour or so. It is not clear whether this exacerbation of his psychotic symptoms is related to the stress of the family arguments, or whether he has been abusing cannabis again, or failing to take his tablets over the weekend. The following additional treatments are likely to be beneficial:

A. individual exploratory psychotherapy
B. family work aimed at increasing the amount of 'expressed emotion' experienced by the patient at home
C. supportive psychotherapy
D. counselling the patient regarding the risks of acute toxic psychosis with cannabis
E. occupational therapy
F. maintenance antipsychotic medication

Support and education are vital components of every treatment plan. The patient must be made aware of the risks of continuing to take cannabis as before. An occupational therapy programme tailored to the patient's strengths and needs is likely to help him to regain confidence and also possibly to acquire new skills. The heated family arguments, and mother's frequent visits while he is in hospital, suggest that the family may be hostile or critical as well as over-involved—all features associated with 'high expressed emotion' families. Lowering the level of expressed emotion by working with the family might reduce the risk of relapse. Exploratory psychotherapy is likely to exacerbate his symptoms rather than improve them.

The discharge diagnosis is schizophrenia, exacerbated by abuse of cannabis. He is discharged on maintenance antipsychotic drug treatment, with an early appointment for the outpatient clinic. FFTTTT

Clinical Case 4

Patient 4

John O, a 23-year-old single man, is brought to casualty by ambulance. The ambulancemen inform the casualty sister that it was John himself who summoned them by dialling 999 and told them on their arrival that he had taken an overdose. The ambulancemen hand over to sister two drug bottles they had picked up from the floor of John's flat. One is labelled 'Amitriptyline', the other 'Temazepam'. Both bottles have John's name on the prescription and both are empty. In casualty, John himself appears quite drowsy but is able to walk with minimal support and to lift himself on to an examination couch. Sister has noted that his breath smells of alcohol.

Immediate priorities in management include:

A. physical examination
B. gathering further information about the overdose
C. assessment of suicidal intent
D. giving prophylactic phenytoin to prevent withdrawal seizures
E. blood gases to check for respiratory alkylosis

John's level of consciousness is the first thing to establish, together with an assessment of his overall physical condition and his potential needs for resuscitation. Temazepam and other benzodiazepines may cause respiratory depression. All tricyclic antidepressants are cardiotoxic. It is therefore good clinical practice to place patients suspected of taking overdoses of tricyclic antidepressants on cardiac monitors. In addition to direct cardiotoxic effects, the anticholinergic effects of the tricyclic antidepressants cause tachycardia and decrease conduction time through the atrioventricular node. Arrhythmias also occur.

At this stage also, it is important to gather as many details as possible of the overdose itself, to plan John's immediate medical care. Patients themselves are sometimes unreliable historians under these circumstances, especially when, as in John's case, they have consumed alcohol as well as an overdose of drugs. Where possible, another informant should be sought. If the overdose was recent (the usual rule of thumb is within four hours of presentation) a stomach wash-out is worth considering. If the delay is longer than this, a stomach wash-out is unlikely to have much effect on the quantity of the drug absorbed (although it is worth remembering that ingestion of large quantities of drugs with anticholinergic effects, such as tricyclic antidepressants or antipsychotic medications, may delay gastric emptying).

Further management will depend on the particular drugs taken in overdose. If there is any uncertainty over this, blood should be obtained for drug screening, particularly for salicylates and paracetamol. If detected in the blood, either of these may require specific treatment, depending on levels obtained. Salicylates in overdose cause respiratory alkalosis, but blood gases to monitor this would normally only be considered if there was clinical and/or laboratory evidence for toxic salicylate levels in the blood.

Further administration of drugs, including anticonvulsants, should be avoided if possible, at least until the patient is alert and oriented and his physical state stable. Exceptions to this are the treatments necessary for overdoses of particular drugs, such as forced alkaline diuresis. TTTFF

Although his speech is slurred, John is well oriented and able to attend to the interview. John states that he felt quite cheerful earlier in the day. He had gone out to lunch with his girlfriend, whom he had only recently met. They had not seen each other for some days and both apparently looked forward to meeting. John had had several pints of lager before they met up, to boost his confidence. They had more alcohol to drink with their lunch. After lunch, he returned home and his girlfriend went back to work. On the way home, John felt that he had created a poor impression and by the time he arrived home, he felt quite desperate that he would not see his girlfriend again. After drinking a few more cans of lager, he spotted the bottles of tablets and quickly swallowed them all. Each bottle apparently contained one week's supply of drugs. He made no effort to lock himself in his bedsit before taking the overdose. On direct questioning, John insists that he has no idea why he took the tablets. Within minutes of taking them, he realised what he had done and telephoned for an ambulance. He is relieved to be in hospital.

John says that he has taken two previous overdoses, within a few weeks of each other, shortly after leaving home five years ago. Further questioning reveals that he has been under some stress recently. He moved to his present bedsit four weeks ago and feels isolated there. He has started a job as a nightwatchman but finds difficulty catching up with his sleep during the day because the neighbourhood is noisy. Before he managed to find the job, he had felt quite desperate and went to see his (new) general practitioner, who prescribed temazepam at night plus amitriptyline 50 mg daily. At the time he saw his general practitioner, John said he was very anxious and also tearful at times and had lost interest in some of his usual activities. However, further questioning reveals no recent features of depression, nor any other specific mental state abnormalities. Although he has consumed a considerable amount of alcohol before arriving in casualty, he denies any features of alcohol dependence.

John remains able to keep awake and attend to the interview. He seems apologetic for having caused so much trouble and asks to be allowed to go home.

The ECG trace is noted to show some prolongation of PR and QT intervals.

A. this overdose shows evidence of suicidal intent
B. the risk of suicide is greater for him than for other men of his age and social status
C. he should be admitted immediately to a psychiatric unit
D. if he refuses a stomach wash-out, he should be placed under the Mental Health Act
E. if he insists on discharging himself, he could be placed under the Mental Health Act to prevent him from doing so
F. he is less likely to have overdosed had the general practitioner given him a higher dose of amitriptyline to begin with

From the evidence elicited so far, there is nothing to suggest that the overdose involved serious suicidal intent. It was impulsive not premeditated, no effort was made to avoid discovery, and he himself summoned help. He shows several suicide risk factors—he is single and isolated, and in addition, has taken two overdoses in the past. This makes him more likely than other men of his age to take further overdoses which may lead to death (possibly unintentionally). As there is no evidence that he is clinically depressed, the dose of his amitriptyline is unlikely to be relevant to his overdose. Had he shown evidence of a depressive illness on admission, one might then consider whether 50 mg amitriptyline at night was an adequate dose—this dose is smaller than that commonly used in psychiatric practice but there is evidence that patients seen in general practice with depression do sometimes respond adequately to such a dose.

Management at this stage should include a stomach wash-out then overnight admission to continue monitoring his ECG and level of consciousness. Because it is his physical state which needs particular observation, it is not appropriate to admit him to a psychiatric unit. Although he remains awake and fairly alert, the ECG abnormalities (widening of the PR and QT intervals) are characteristic of overdose with tricyclic antidepressants.

The Mental Health Act does allow for John to be detained in hospital for further assessment, if he refuses to be admitted voluntarily. However, no evidence has been elicited that John has a mental disorder—this is one criterion necessary to admit him on a section. The expression of suicidal intent is not necessarily indicative of a mental disorder. However, if clinical judgement suggested that the patient's suicidal intent was a feature of a psychiatric disorder, then it would be appropriate to offer the patient voluntary admission and, if he refused, to consider using the Act to detain him.

The Mental Health Act is of no help if he refuses a stomach wash-out, as the Act is confined in its applications to the assessment and management of mental disorder. Technically, performing a stomach wash-out without the patient's consent could be interpreted as assault. Equally, failure to treat when it is essential to do so may be seen as negligent. However, under common law, treatments may be administered without consent if they are urgently necessary and if without them there is a considerable risk of death or serious illness. In John's case, it is likely that he has taken relatively few tablets. Provided that he agrees to admission, there is probably no need to insist on a stomach wash-out. FTFFTF

John agrees to remain in hospital voluntarily and is admitted to the short-stay ward overnight. The following morning, his physical observations are stable and reveal no abnormalities. He complains of a headache but is otherwise reasonably cheerful. He says he is puzzled by what happened the previous day and cannot understand why he took the overdose. He shows no evidence of depression and denies any ideas of suicide.

In a further interview, he tells you that he is the eldest of three siblings, with one sister at University studying psychology and the other doing 'A' levels. His father is an intelligent man, a physicist who eventually became a teacher.

Having stayed at home to look after the children when they were small, mother subsequently did a part-time degree course in sociology. After getting his 'O' levels, John himself failed to continue his studies and 'dropped out', much to his parents' disapproval. He describes how, in his family, success was always equated with academic achievements. Friction between his parents and himself eventually led to his leaving home. After 'drifting' for a time, John decided to take himself in hand and found his present bedsit and his job. He has always felt rather lacking in self-confidence, particularly in his relationships. He has had three girlfriends previously, but these relationships only lasted a few months at most.

A. he should be admitted to a psychiatric unit
B. even if he showed clear features of a depressive illness, he must not be discharged on amitriptyline
C. he should be discharged on a different antidepressant
D. the only appropriate follow-up for him is at a psychiatric clinic
E. in the longer term, he may be a candidate for psychotherapy
F. he should be advised to abstain from alcohol

John clearly does not need to remain in hospital. Keeping someone like John in hospital at this stage may do more harm than good. Being in hospital encourages patients to view themselves as ill, and often to relinquish to staff all responsibility for getting themselves better. While this may be appropriate for someone who is, for example, acutely psychotic, the same does not apply to someone like John. However, this does not mean that follow-up is unnecessary. There is no one intervention suitable for all patients admitted after overdose—what is offered should be tailored to the individual's needs. Who follows up the patient will depend also on local resources. If the patient is psychiatrically ill (but does not require inpatient care), follow-up in a psychiatric out-patient clinic is appropriate. In John's case, there is no convincing evidence of a psychiatric illness and he might therefore be followed up by a social worker rather than a psychiatrist. There is no need to prescribe further antidepressants. At the time he presented to his general practitioner, he may have appeared clinically depressed, but in retrospect his course over the few weeks preceding his admission was not that of a depressive illness. If he was depressed, the choice of antidepressants would depend on the likelihood of his taking a further overdose. Not all depressed people feel suicidal and it might therefore be appropriate to continue with amitriptyline. Some of the newer antidepressants are safer than amitriptyline and the tricyclics in overdose, but if it was likely that a depressed patient would take a further overdose, admission to a psychiatric unit should be considered. Given that this is John's third overdose, many psychiatrists would not take the risk of further overdoses with amitriptyline. However, this decision will depend on a thorough assessment in each individual case.

Although John's overdose was associated (as is quite common) with taking alcohol, no evidence has been elicited of alcohol abuse or dependence. It is thus inappropriate to advise him to abstain from alcohol, although counselling about the effects of alcohol would probably be helpful.

From John's story, it is evident that he has a low self-image and difficulties with relationships with his peers. It is also likely that problems exist between himself and his family. It might be possible to address some of these issues in psychotherapy, either individual or group. However, many psychotherapists would be wary of taking a patient on for exploratory psychotherapy who has a history of several overdoses. This suggests that he might not have the capacity to work through the stresses of a therapeutic relationship and that therapy could precipitate a further overdose when it becomes stressful. However, problems such as John's often show a good response to cognitive therapy. Whoever offers John follow-up appointments in the short term after his discharge could assess his suitability and motivation for psychotherapy. FFFFTF

Patient 5

An 18-year-old single woman complains of amenorrhoea. She has been admitted to a gynaecology ward, where investigations fail to find a gynaecological cause for her amenorrhoea. Psychiatric assessment is requested.

The patient states that she experienced menarch at the age of 13 years. Her cycles were irregular until 15 years and then became regular until six months ago when they ceased. It had been noticed on admission that she was underweight and the nurses had noticed that she ate very little on the ward and that her mother had brought in a supply of 'diet foods' to sustain her. She shows no concern about her weight and avoids 'fattening' foods.

On the ward she is lying in bed reading 'Jane Fonda's Workout'. She is of average height and obviously thin with cyanotic extremities and slight enlargement of her parotid salivary glands. Her weight is 6½ stones (41 kg).

The following findings are likely on taking a history and carrying out a physical and mental state examination:

A. denial of thinness
B. claims of adequate dietary intake
C. lanugo hair
D. bradycardia
E. avitaminosis
F. deranged urea and electrolytes
G. raised plasma thyroxine
H. self-induced vomiting
I. laxative abuse
J. morbid fear of fatness

In any young female with unexplained weight loss and amenorrhoea the diagnosis of anorexia nervosa should be entertained. These patients exhibit a characteristic psychopathology which includes a morbid fear of fatness, a relentless pursuit of thinness and a distorted body image, such that they tend to overestimate body size. Often there is denial of illness and patients may claim adequate dietary intake.

A number of physical signs secondary to chronic undernutrition may occur including the growth of fine lanugo hair, bradycardia and cyanotic extremities. In spite of undernutrition, avitaminosis is rare. About one-third or more give a history of self-induced vomiting or laxative abuse as a means of weight reduction, and if this is severe, electrolyte disturbances may occur. Thyroid function may be reduced, with a low plasma thyroxine (T4). TTTTFTFTTT

The history reveals that she is single and living with her parents. Father is a business executive who frequently travels abroad and mother is an attractive but dissatisfied housewife. Eighteen months ago the patient weighed 8¾ stones (54 kg). Twelve months ago, a month before her 'A' levels, she went on a diet 'to please my boyfriend' and found that she enjoyed the feeling of slimming and 'being good'. Over the next six months, her weight declined to 7 stones (44 kg) and her periods ceased. Her 'A' level results were disappointing and her illness prevented her from taking up a place at university. She had ended a two-year relationship, which had not been a sexual one, four months previously and was hoping to obtain employment at a local health and beauty centre. She has a brother two years her senior who is studying psychology at university and who feels strongly that there is a physical cause for her condition. She reports having been concerned about her weight in her early teens but has never dieted to the same extent before.

She admits that she may have allowed her dieting to go too far and claims she would now like to gain weight. Her mother reports however that she appears terrified of gaining weight and suspects she is hiding food and surreptitiously inducing vomiting. Relationships at home are strained and her parents argue about who is to blame for not inducing her to eat more.

The following statements are likely to be true:

A. the diagnosis is anorexia nervosa
B. the diagnosis is bulimia nervosa
C. hypopituitarism needs exclusion
D. thyrotoxicosis is likely
E. a CAT brain scan is mandatory
F. she may have demineralised teeth
G. she requires urgent transfer to the psychiatric unit
H. the condition is secondary to parental disharmony

The diagnosis is almost certainly anorexia nervosa. She demonstrates the characteristic psychopathology, and she has lost more than 20% of her healthy body weight and is amenorrhoeic. Although she may induce vomiting, she has none of the other features of bulimia nervosa. Demineralised teeth (found in some patients with bulimia) are thus possible but unlikely. Physical causes of weight loss and amenorrhoea such as hypopituitarism, thyrotoxicosis or tuberculosis are most unlikely, but should be excluded with appropriate investigations. CAT brain scan will sometimes reveal non-specific changes but is not warranted unless physical examination suggests an intracranial lesion. Admission to a psychiatric unit is only required when the weight loss is acute or dangerously low. If the weight is less than 35–40 kg in the average patient, urgent admission to a unit specialising in the treatment of eating disorders should be arranged, otherwise outpatient treatment should be attempted first. Although there is evidence of marital disharmony at present this could be secondary to the disorder in the patient. TFTFFTFF

The patient is interviewed with her parents the following week. They report that they are at the end of their tether. Their daughter will not increase her food consumption and exercises excessively. They fear for her safety and are critical of her having 'ruined her career'. Mother dominates the interview and father seems preoccupied and somewhat depressed. The patient herself denies any serious problem and accuses her parents and doctor of excessive concern.

Having taken a full history and discussed the situation with the family, what action would be appropriate?

A. admit her to the psychiatric unit
B. negotiate a sensible diet under parental supervision
C. administer tricyclic antidepressants
D. see her regularly in the outpatient department with a view to admission if her weight falls further
E. request that she keep an accurate diary of her food consumption

Unless her weight continues to decline to a dangerous extent, outpatient treatment should be attempted first. The patient is asked to keep a diary of her dietry intake and a sensible diet is negotiated. An agreement can be made to involve the parents in her refeeding schedule. Antidepressants have little value unless depressive symptoms are prominent. She should be seen frequently and an accurate record of her weight be kept and discussed with the patient and her family. Some experts prefer a family-oriented approach from the outset and there is evidence that younger patients with a short history do better with family therapy than with individual treatment in which the family is not directly involved. FTFTT

She is seen weekly and her weight remains stable at 6¾ stones (42 kg). She claims to be eating 'normally' but inspection of her diary reveals that she is consuming approximately 1200 Kcals/day mainly in the form of 'diet foods'. She now admits to self-induced vomiting but adds that the frequency of this has reduced from twice daily to twice weekly.

The following are likely to be aetiologically important:

A. anxieties about separation from her family
B. fears of sexuality
C. brain tumour
D. high expectations of achievement

The aetiology of anorexia nervosa is unknown. Some experts have emphasised separation from the family as an important stressor. This patient's illness started in the setting of discussions about a planned move away from home to university. Fears of womanhood and the growing threat of sexuality have been implicated by other authors. This patient may have feared her boyfriend's growing sexual interest, and she rejected him in the course of this illness. She comes from a high-achieving family and the added stress of her examinations and future university career may have contributed. TTFT

Over the next few months she begins to eat more and her weight increases to 7¼ stones (46 kg). She begins to relate to the doctor in a more mature way and talks with great anxiety about her father, who she believes is overworked and depressed. She fears he will suffer a 'heart attack' like her uncle who had died two months before her 'A' levels. She also reports that since the onset of her own illness, her father had curtailed his business trips and her parents had seen much more of each other. She fears that if she went to university, her parents' marriage could break down or her father suffer a 'heart attack'.

Further management should include:

A. ongoing behavioural methods to increase her dietry intake
B. regular follow-up with attention to her weight
C. supportive psychotherapy
D. family therapy
E. at least six months' treatment with an antidepressant

This patient should be followed up with attention to her weight and eating habits until she is relaxed about her weight and is eating freely. Normally a target should be set close to her premorbid weight and return of menstrual function can be anticipated, especially if the history has been relatively short. Supportive psychotherapy should be provided to help her to relinquish her 'sick role'. Family therapy would also be an appropriate treatment option, particularly in view of her age and the relatively short history. There is no evidence that antidepressants alter the course of the illness. TTTTF

One year after presentation her weight is 9 stone (57 kg) and she is menstruating regularly. She eats three meals a day, although at times of stress she tends to reduce her food intake. She no longer induces vomiting or takes laxatives. Father has moved to another department which does not involve travel abroad and the family atmosphere appears much improved. Her parents appear ready for her to separate from the family and she has applied for a course in veterinary science in another town.

The following statements are true:

A. she has a relatively poor prognosis compared with other anorexics
B. the final diagnosis is bulimia nervosa
C. the condition was caused by parental disharmony
D. there may be recurrences at times of stress
E. she is unlikely to complete her course

Approximately one-third of patients will recover after a single episode of anorexia nervosa, while about one half will go on to develop a chronic disorder with incomplete recovery or relapses and remissions. The most important good prognostic sign is a history of less than 18 months duration. This applies in the present case and, together with the fact that she is now maintaining her weight at a healthy level, suggests a relatively good outlook. Nevertheless, it is possible that she may relapse, particularly at times of stress, especially if she leaves the parental home before domestic conflicts are resolved.

The most likely formulation in this case is that conflicts concerning the transition from dependency to independence, with its associated threats of sexuality, were important. Concerns about the parental relationship and father's health made it difficult to leave home, especially after the death of her paternal uncle. The importance of high achievement in this family may also have been contributory. Although parental disharmony is evident, this could have been aggravated or even produced by the stress of having an anorexic daughter. All this is speculative, but can be used in psychotherapy. Although there is a risk of relapse, the indications in this patient are that she is likely to complete her course, especially with ongoing counselling. FFFTF

Clinical Case 6

Patient 6

Miss T, a 68-year-old woman who lives alone, is brought to the casualty department by ambulance at 10.30 p.m. Immediately before her arrival a doctor unfamiliar with Miss T's background telephones the casualty department to inform the receiving casualty officer of the circumstances prompting his referral of Miss T to the hospital. He had been called by one of Miss T's neighbours after the neighbour had noted that Miss T had burns on her legs which seemed to have become infected. The neighbour had taken a benevolent interest in Miss T since her last discharge from hospital some 18 months previously and was concerned that she was spending a lot of time in the pub and neglecting herself physically. The ambulancemen report that Miss T had been initially agreeable to visiting the hospital but had subsequently attempted to jump out of the ambulance while it was on the road and had made statements that the police were trying to burn her house down. They also report that she had been incontinent of urine.

Immediate steps in Miss T's further management should include:

A. administration of diazepam 10 mg i.v. to sedate her
B. examination of her cognitive state
C. complete physical examination
D. transfer to the psychiatric ward for evaluation
E. blood chemistry, haematology, chest X-ray and urine analysis

The immediate aim is to ascertain the basis of Miss T's disturbed mental state and in particular to exclude serious physical illness. Sedation should be avoided if at all possible as the depression of consciousness which it induces may considerably impede clinical assessment and indeed may precipitate respiratory depression and coma if conscious state is already impaired.

Examination of the cognitive state is essential—in particular, simple clinical testing of orientation, attention and concentration and short-term memory. These aspects of the clinical examination may be overlooked when the patient's behaviour appears obviously to be governed by psychotic thinking but they must be undertaken to exclude an underlying organic cerebral or systemic disorder. In Miss T's case the presence of possibly infected burns, a history of incontinence, self-neglect and alcohol abuse provide further pointers to a possible organic aetiology.

A full physical examination to exclude both neurological and systemic pathology is also required. Especially in the elderly, psychiatric disorder often has often multifactorial causes, and a cursory examination may fail to discover all of the contributory pathologies. Physical examination should be supplemented by appropriate physical investigations depending on the history and findings at examination. In Miss T's case, blood chemistry, haematology, chest X-ray and urine analysis are the essential minimum in view of the clinical feature suggestive of an organic aetiology.

Although Miss T's claims that the police are trying to burn down her house appear bizarre and possibly psychotic and her behaviour in trying to jump out of the ambulance dangerous, these, are not in themselves indications for immediate assessment in the psychiatry ward. Virtually all psychiatric symptoms may arise out of organic cerebral or systemic disorders and in such cases the first priority is to identify and treat the underlying disorder which in some cases may be life-threatening. FTTFT

On cognitive state examination Miss T is drowsy, disoriented in time and place, has severely impaired concentration, and testing of short-term memory proves impossible. Her speech is at times incoherent but she reiterates several times that the police and now also the hospital staff are intent on burning her house down and claims that she can see snakes on top of her bedclothes. She continually claws at the curtains around her bed and at times appears to be talking loudly even though nobody else is with her.

Physical examination reveals some dehydration, a slight fever, tachycardia, mild hypertension and profuse sweatiness. There is a bilateral hand tremor, left lateral rectus palsy and nystagmus. The liver is enlarged and tender and spider naevi are visible on the abdominal wall. Infected second-degree burns are present on both thighs.

Laboratory investigations confirm moderate dehydration and reveal a raised aspartate transaminase, a mild normochromic normocytic anaemia and a polymorphonuclear leukocytosis. Chest X-ray and urinalysis are unremarkable.

The following are indicated:

A. immediate insertion of 5% dextrose drip
B. a likely presumptive diagnosis of senile dementia of the Alzheimer type
C. administration of intravenous thiamine
D. administration of a reducing regime of chlormethiazole
E. early consultation with the old age psychiatry team in order to plan for a long-stay psychiatric bed

The clinical features point to an acute brain syndrome, with impairment of consciousness, other cognitive deficits and probable visual hallucinations. The history of probable alcohol abuse obtained from her neighbour, together with clinical signs of liver disease and withdrawal phenomena such as tremor and profuse sweatiness, indicate a diagnosis of delirium tremens. Additional neurological signs including left lateral rectus palsy and nystagmus are also present. These signs indicate an additional diagnosis of Wernicke's encephalopathy, which may be confirmed by finding elevated blood pyruvate levels. Mild anaemia and infected burns may also be contributory factors to her mental state. Multiple pathologies in Miss T's case highlight the need for thorough examination in all cases of acute brain syndrome. The diagnosis of dementia cannot be made in the presence of an acute brain syndrome unless there is firm evidence of dementia preceding the acute disturbances associated with the impairment of consciousness. In most cases acute brain syndromes resolve fully when the underlying causes are treated and there is no reason at this stage of Miss T's management to be planning long-stay psychiatric care.

Management is directed towards treatment of the underlying causes. Delirium tremens may be controlled by a reducing regime of chlormethiazole. This drug is preferable to the antipsychotic drugs commonly employed for sedation in acute brain syndromes in view of its anticonvulsant properties. Epileptic fits may complicate alcohol withdrawal and occasionally necessitate additional anticonvulsant medication. Rehydration and the maintenance of electrolyte balance are also necessary. Immediate administration of 5% dextrose however is contraindicated in the presence of Wernicke's encephalopathy as this leads to further metabolism of the depleted thiamine store. Normal saline should be used initially if an intravenous infusion is required for rehydration. Intravenous administration of thiamine is urgently required to prevent irreversible deterioration to Korsakoff's psychosis. Treatment of the infected burns and investigation and treatment of the anaemia will also need to be undertaken. FFTTF

After assessment and immediate treatment in the casualty department, Miss T is transferred to a medical ward. She becomes progressively more alert and coherent. Her ideas of persecution by the police disappear and she is felt by the nursing staff to be an amiable but rather vague elderly lady. However, the nurses note that she has difficulty in dressing and also, at times, in finding words to express herself. She is incontinent of urine at night. She sometimes loses her way around the ward and cannot always find her way back to her own bed.

In a further assessment, one month after her admission, the following are indicated:

A. a further clinical assessment of her cognitive state
B. psychometric testing
C. a presumptive diagnosis of Korsakoff's psychosis
D. occupational therapy assessment
E. an EEG as an essential investigation

The persistence of incontinence together with her difficulties in dressing and problems in word-finding indicate that, despite resolution of her acute brain syndrome, there are residual cognitive deficits in cognitive function, indicating an additional chronic pathology. Korsakoff's psychosis involves a disorder of memory with relative preservation of other cognitive functions. This is not consistent with the nurses' observations, which suggest the presence of dysphasia and dyspraxia.

Her current cognitive deficits require further investigation, in particular to establish whether they are diffuse (as is characteristic of dementia) or focal, and to identify reversible causes. Thorough clinical cognitive testing is essential, together with formal psychometric assessment. An EEG may be helpful, in that focal pathology sometimes gives focal EEG abnormalities, although the absence of such focal changes on the EEG does not exclude focal brain damage. A CAT brain scan would possibly be more useful.

The effects of Miss T's cognitive deficits on her daily living activities will also need to be assessed. This information, crucial in planning for her longer-term care, cannot be gleaned from the results of cognitive testing. Occupational therapy assessment, first in hospital and then at Miss T's home, will enable abilities of self-care, cooking, shopping and other personal skills to be determined, on the basis of which further support in hospital and/or the community can be planned. TTFTF

Further assessment reveals that, given a name and address to remember, she is able to recall 7 out of 8 items immediately but only 3 items after 5 minutes. She is unable to name the present prime minister or monarch, but correctly identifies that the monarch is female and has four children, although unable to remember any of their names correctly. She is able to name correctly a pen, a coat, a key and a door but not a belt buckle, a cuff-link or a watch strap. However, she is able to describe accurately and in detail how to get from her home to numerous other places by public transport, and demonstrates a clear knowledge of numerous bus routes. She is able to copy a circle and triangle drawn by the doctor, but has great difficulty copying a cube. Asked to draw a clock face, she has difficulty placing the numbers accurately. She declines to do serial sevens but says that 9 from 30 equals 4. She has difficulty in rapidly touching her thumb with each of her fingers, worse with her left hand than the right. She also makes mistakes in telling left from right. She is unable to identify a £1 coin by sight and, with her eyes closed, cannot identify a key by touch.

The CAT brain scan reveals generalised cortical atrophy with widened sulci but also several small focal areas on the lateral aspect of both hemispheres, consistent with previous infarcts.

On the basis of these results:

A. the most likely diagnosis is dementia
B. her ability to remember bus routes is an unexpected finding, given the other results
C. her ability to recall local geography and bus routes indicates that her deficits are focal and argue against this being Alzheimer-type dementia
D. the CAT scan is inconsistent with Alzheimer-type dementia as the diagnosis
E. these results indicate that she is very unlikely to be able to cope successfully at home
F. that she can recall 7 of 8 items of a name and address immediately is against her having any significant memory deficit

She clearly has memory deficits. The fact that she can correctly recall 7 of 8 items of a name and address immediately after hearing them is an important part of this test, indicating that she has registered the address in memory. Without this observation, her limited recall after 5 minutes would be impossible to interpret. It is not uncommon for some aspects of memory to be preserved in someone with dementia (whether Alzheimer-type or multi-infarct), and her ability to recall bus routes is thus not inconsistent with the diagnosis of Alzheimer-type dementia.

In addition to her memory deficits, she demonstrates numerous other impairments, both cognitive and neurological. She demonstrates nominal dysphasia (demonstrated best when patients are asked to name relatively uncommonly used words), difficulties with simple arithmetic, visuospatial agnosia, tactile agnosia, left–right disorientation and dyspraxia. This indicates that her impairments are not focal but involve diffuse parts of the brain. Hence the diagnosis is dementia.

Although there are focal changes in the CAT scan, there is also diffuse atropy. This does not preclude Alzheimer-type dementia as the diagnosis, and it may be that both Alzheimer-type and multi-infarct dementia contribute to the overall clinical picture. Further details of her behaviour at home over the months prior to her admission might clarify this—a gradual (though possibly subtle) deterioration in cognitive function would point to Alzheimer-type dementia, as would a positive family history. Details of her previous hospital admission (reason for admission and level of functioning at that time) would help to clarify this.

Except where cognitive impairments are extreme, it is unwise to try to predict how adequately a patient might cope at home from formal clinical assessment alone. Miss T appeared to function well at home until recently, is probably still able to find her way about without getting lost, and has the benefit of a supportive neighbour. Occupational therapy assessment, preferably with a home visit, is important. TFFFFF

Patient 7

Michael P, a 34-year-old man, married for seven years, complains that for the last three years, he has been unable to maintain an erection sufficient for vaginal penetration during intercourse, and that he ejaculates either before or at the moment of penetration. His wife has been his only sexual partner since they were married, and their sexual relationship was previously satisfactory.

Which of the following diagnoses apply?

A. primary erectile impotence
B. secondary erectile impotence
C. premature ejaculation
D. ejaculatory incompetence
E. low libido

He suffers from premature ejaculation. In addition, he has erectile impotence. He has not always had erectile impotence, as his sexual relationship with his wife was satisfactory until three years ago. Thus this is secondary rather than primary erectile impotence. FTTFF

He is physically healthy and a non-smoker, but drinks one or two single measures of whisky most evenings. He has suffered from a peptic ulcer in the past and is currently taking cimetidine 400 mg twice daily. He works as an accountant investigating fraud for the Inland Revenue Service.

Which of the following factors are likely to be contributing to his problems:

A. cimetidine treatment
B. effects of alcohol
C. other organic factors
D. age
E. stress at work
F. psychological factors in the marital relationship

Sexual dysfunction in a 34-year-old man cannot be explained in terms of age. Erectile impotence can result from excessive consumption of alcohol, but his reported consumption hardly qualifies as excessive and there is no reason to doubt his account in this case. Alcohol is more likely to lead to ejaculatory failure than to premature ejaculation. This combination of erectile impotence and premature ejaculation is more likely to be due to psychological factors like difficulties in the marital relationship and stress at work. A number of organic problems may cause sexual dysfunction, including diabetes, renal failure, Addison's disease and thyroid dysfunction. Investigations should be carried out as indicated by the presentation of each individual case. In Mr. P's case, he is physically healthy, making it unlikely that his sexual problems would be completely accounted for by organic factors. However, impotence is a rare but recognised effect of cimetidine. The drug is stopped but there is no improvement. TFFFTT

His wife agrees to be interviewed. She is 32 years old and is a highly paid, successful banker with a foreign bank. Her work often takes her abroad for short trips. She works long hours. Her interests are interior decorating and expensive clothes. The couple have no children and they are undecided about whether or not to start a family at present. The wife has an intra-uterine device as their only form of contraception. She does not consider that they have a serious sexual problem. She can reach orgasm with self-stimulation but has never done so with intercourse alone. The couple have sex about once a month and she finds this perfectly acceptable, although her husband feels that this is too infrequent. She fears that her husband has difficulty coping with her career success. She also denies any sexual liaison outside the marriage.

The following diagnoses apply to the wife:

A. primary anorgasmia
B. low sexual interest
C. vaginismus
D. dyspareunia
E. no sexual problem

She appears to have low sexual interest and a coital orgasmic problem. A woman with primary anorgasmia has never achieved orgasm, which is not the case here. There are no features in the history of vaginismus or dyspareunia. FTFFF

Which of the following factors are likely to be important in the genesis of this couple's sexual problems:

A. fear of pregnancy
B. hormonal changes during the wife's menstrual cycle
C. tiredness on the wife's part
D. unresolved issues in the couple's relationship
E. the husband's sense of inadequacy in the relationship

Tiredness and changes in sexual desire with the menstrual cycle would not produce the complaints described. Fear of pregnancy is a common cause of sexual dysfunction, and may be important in this case, even though Mrs P uses effective contraception. Sexual difficulties often reflect more general problems within a relationship. In this case, it is possible that Mrs P has rather overshadowed her husband in her career—any effects of this on the relationship are unlikely to have been acknowledged by either partner. TFFTT

Mrs P admits that there may be problems with their sexual and marital relationship, but initially rejects treatment, being convinced that the couple can solve their difficulties without outside help. However, they return after three months, as the situation has deteriorated. The first-line treatment options to be considered at this stage include:

A. individual psychotherapy for the husband
B. individual psychotherapy for the wife
C. directive marital and sex therapy
D. group therapy for Mrs P in a group for women with orgasmic dysfunction
E. some counselling sessions to provide support for the couple

Conjoint marital and sex therapy, a form of behavioural psychotherapy, would be the most effective treatment for this couple's problems. Simple support for the couple is unlikely to succeed. The difficulties clearly affect both partners in the relationship, and are best addressed in conjoint sessions, involving both husband and wife. Suggesting that Mrs P might join a group for women with orgasmic dysfunction might be worth considering at a later stage but not immediately, especially as focusing on Mrs P's difficulty in achieving orgasm during intercourse might make Mr P even more anxious about his sexual performance. FFTFF

The couple agree to a series of time-limited sessions with a trained sex and marital therapist, which Mr and Mrs P will attend together. Initially, the treatment might usefully include:

A. testosterone for Mrs P
B. testosterone for Mr P
C. the 'squeeze' technique
D. undertaking to have sexual intercourse at least once a week
E. sensate focus exercises
F. facilitating communication of feelings and emotions between the partners
G. a penile prosthesis for Mr P

The treatment involves a graded series of 'homework' tasks. To begin with, these involve sensate focus exercises, in which the couple practise arousing each other sexually, each focusing on the other's arousal rather than his or her own, and being guided by the other partner to discover what the partner finds particularly stimulating sexually. An important part of this treatment involves encouraging the sharing of feelings, in particular for each partner to tell the other what he or she finds arousing and pleasurable. These exercises begin with a complete ban on genital contact and sexual intercourse. Subsequently genital contact is reintroduced, and once the couple are more confident of reaching this stage without major difficulties, sexual intercourse may be resumed.

The 'squeeze' technique might be used specifically for Mr P's premature ejaculation. Taking testosterone sometimes (but not always) helps in those cases where a man's sexual dysfunction is related particularly to low testosterone levels, but there is no reason to suspect that this applies in Mr P's case. Giving testosterone to Mrs P is also unlikely to be beneficial. A penile prosthesis may be indicated where erectile failure is due to an organic cause, such as diabetes or renal failure. This also does not apply in Mr P's case. FFTFTTF

Mr and Mrs P attend regularly for ten sessions. They report on their progress with the graded exercises, and any difficulties they have found with the exercises are explored in dicussion with the therapist. After the ten sessions, which of the following would be reasonable expectations of outcome:

A. Mrs P experiences orgasm with intercourse alone on most occasions
B. Mr P shows improved control of his premature ejaculation
C. Mr P has a complete return of his erectile function

D. an increase in Mrs P's libido
E. more open communication and expression of feelings between the two partners

After ten sessions, a considerable improvement in the couple's problems can be expected, but it is unlikely that their problems will have gone completely. The therapy is likely to have improved their ability to share their feelings, which might be expected to have effects beyond their sexual relationship. FTFTT

Patient 8

Mrs Ivy P is a 68-year-old widow, living alone in a first-floor flat. Her downstairs neighbour has contacted the Social Services Department because, for the past two days, water has been seeping through her ceiling, apparently from Ivy's flat. Ivy will not open the door to the neighbour, but tells her neighbour, through the letterbox, to go away and leave her alone. The social workers have no record of previous contact with Ivy. One of them attempts to visit, but is again told through the letterbox to 'mind her own business'. One of Ivy's neighbours tells the social worker that Ivy has been behaving rather oddly for some weeks and that she had complained to the police that her neighbours were trying to harm her. The neighbour thinks Ivy gets on quite well with her general practitioner, who was very supportive after the death two years previously of Ivy's husband.

The social worker requests a domiciliary visit by a psychiatrist. She also contacts the general practitioner, but he is away on a half-day. The psychiatrist can find no previous record of Ivy attending the psychiatric department. The psychiatrist and social worker arrive at Ivy's flat to find the keyhole of her front door stuffed with cotton wool. Ivy refuses to answer the door but shouts at them to be left alone, adding, 'It's those people downstairs—they're out to get me—and you're all in this together. It's all your fault.'

Based on the information so far available, the most likely diagnoses are:

A. depression
B. paraphrenia
C. acute brain syndrome
D. dementia

The evidence so far indicates that Ivy's behaviour appears to have changed recently. She has become hostile and her comments to the police as well as the psychiatrist suggest that she may have persecutory delusions. Any one of the diagnoses listed could produce such a picture in someone of her age. However, dementia and paraphrenia are the most likely. That Ivy has been noted to be behaving oddly for some weeks is against an acute brain syndrome. She appears quite active, despite isolating herself, which suggests that depression is unlikely. Also, rather than blaming herself for what is happening (which is usual in depression), she blames others. FTFT

What options are there for appropriately managing the situation?

A. the psychiatrist should tell Ivy that he'll simply wait outside her door until she agrees to talk to him
B. break the door down
C. call the police to help gain access to Ivy's flat
D. leave and come back tomorrow
E. apply for a Section 135 order
F. contact the general practitioner

Telling Ivy that she will have to open the door eventually is provocative and unlikely to succeed. At this stage, nobody is legally empowered to break into Ivy's flat. However, the social worker can apply for a Section 135. This is a warrant issued by a magistrate, on the basis of information from the social worker, to authorise a policeman to enter a home of other private premises, by force if necessary, to allow the assessment of a person suspected of being mentally disordered and the removal of that person to hospital. Planning a further visit the next day is unlikely to succeed, as there is evidence that Ivy has opened her door to no one for some days. However, it appears that Ivy may have a good relationship with her general practitioner. If she trusts him, it may be possible that he could persuade her to open her door. FFFFTT

The social worker and psychiatrist discuss whether Ivy's present mental state puts her or her neighbours in any immediate danger. They conclude that, although she is clearly distressed by her beliefs, the whole situation appears to have remained static for some days at least and is unlikely to change before the next day. Also, the water coming through into the downstairs flat appears to have stopped and there appears to be no immediate danger from this. Rather than applying for a Section 135, they decide to return the following day with the general practitioner.

The following morning, after a long exchange through her letterbox, Ivy finally allows the general practitioner into her flat and later agrees to talk to the psychiatrist and social worker. She recognises the general practitioner immediately and accurately recalls when they last met at the time of her husband's death.

The flat is in a mess. All the windows are taped shut and furniture is piled up against one of the doors. The pictures have been taken off the walls. Ivy has been sitting in one chair in her living room, surrounded by half-empty packets of biscuits. There is a photograph of a middle-aged man (presumably her late husband, a few years ago) prominently displayed on a little table beside her chair.

Ivy is at first suspicious of her visitors, but relaxes a little when she realises they are interested in knowing what has been happening to her. She says that her neighbours started persecuting her some weeks ago, by passing poisonous gases through her keyhole and through the plumbing system. She says that she tried to 'flush out' the gases by keeping the water running all the time. The neighbours have also planted miniature loudspeakers all over the flat, to torment her by telling her what they're planning to do.

At this stage, which of the following are appropriate?

A. doing a full cognitive assessment
B. avoiding any mention of her late husband, in case mention of him were to upset her too much
C. telling Ivy that she has to come into hospital
D. giving her an intramuscular injection of chlorpromazine
E. reassuring Ivy that the neighbours are not trying to talk to her through loudspeakers

Although some of Ivy's symptoms are now clearer, there is not yet sufficient information to establish a working diagnosis. It is not yet clear what will be the best way of managing her disorder thus starting a management plan (giving chlorpromazine or deciding to admit her to hospital) would be premature. Ivy's belief about the neighbours' loudspeakers is delusional. She is thus unlikely to respond to reassurance, which may even antagonise her if she feels the psychiatrist and social worker do not understand her difficulties. The loss of her husband may be relevant to her present disorder and is in any case an important life event. It is therefore important to talk about this in this interview and elicit Ivy's feelings, even if she does find this upsetting. TFFFF

The differential diagnosis now includes:

A. depression
B. paraphrenia
C. dementia
D. schizophrenia

The most likely diagnoses are paraphrenia and depression. Both can present with persecutory delusions, but these are congruent with mood in depression, and usually not mood-congruent in paraphrenia. Ivy appears to be hallucinating (the 'loudspeakers'), a point in favour of paraphrenia, in which hallucinations are more common than in depression. Hallucinations and delusions also occur in acute and chronic brain syndromes. Formal cognitive testing will help to exclude these, but the fact that she recognised the general practitioner as she did suggests that considerable memory impairment is unlikely. To diagnose schizophrenia confidently, there should (in someone of Ivy's age) be evidence of a past history of psychotic illness—it is unusual for schizophrenia to present for the first time at 68. TTTT

On direct questioning, Ivy admits to having eaten little recently and says her sleep has been poor. She has slept in her chair, as she believes the neighbours have tampered with her bed. She says she keeps herself occupied by listening to her radio—she becomes absorbed with this, and it seems to drown the noise of the loudspeakers. Having had her attention directed to the photograph beside her, she confirms that it is of her husband and becomes tearful, adding that she misses him terribly. She is fully oriented in time and place. She denies the possibility that she might be ill, insisting that the police should be called to arrest her neighbours.
    Conclusions from this are:

A. she has definite biological features of depression
B. there is evidence that she has a morbid grief reaction
C. the fact that she is fully oriented excludes an acute brain syndrome as a
   likely diagnosis

Although she eats poorly, this may be due to her circumstances rather than her appetite—since she has not been out of her flat much recently, and has been surviving on biscuits and other similar foods. Similarly, sleeping in a chair is likely to be uncomfortable. Thus these *might* be symptoms of depression, but they have other possible explanations. The fact that she can become absorbed in listening to the radio argues against the diagnosis of melancholia. Becoming tearful when talking about a spouse who died is not unusual. Neither this, nor having his photograph to hand, are necessarily signs of a morbid grief reaction. Being fully oriented makes the diagnosis of acute brain syndrome less likely, but does not exclude it, as one feature of acute brain syndromes is fluctuation in level of consciousness. FFF

The possible features of melancholia elicited in the interview are unconvincing. The presence of delusions and hallucinations, together with relatively good preservation of the personality, supports the diagnosis of paraphrenia. Bearing in mind that she has already insisted that she is not ill and that this is a matter for the police, appropriate action at this stage would possibly include:

A. telling her that it would be best if she came into hospital
B. asking if she'll agree to take medication
C. placing her on Section 3 of the Mental Health Act
D. placing her on Section 4 of the Mental Health Act
E. starting her on an intramuscular injection of 50 mg fluphenazine decanoate every week

She clearly requires treatment with antipsychotic medication. That she apparently lacks any insight does not mean that she will necessarily refuse admission to hospital. Patients may, as she has done, act on their delusions and deny they are ill and still agree to admission. Whether she is likely to agree to take medication is a crucial question. If she is unlikely to take medication reliably, this strengthens the argument in favour of admission to hospital, under the Mental Health Act if necessary, because without medication, her disorder and her circumstances are likely to deteriorate, placing her (and possibly also the downstairs neighbour) at risk. If she refuses admission, it would be appropriate to admit her under Section 2 for observation, in the first instance. Only when the diagnosis is adequately established is it appropriate to consider a Section 3—a brief first interview is insufficient for this, particularly with no record of any past psychiatric history. Section 4 is an 'emergency' section, for use when only one medical recommendation can be obtained and detention of the patient is urgently necessary. In this case, there are two doctors already present to complete the medical recommendations for Section 2.

  Placing her on a depot injection of an antipsychotic drug is another option to consider. However, because the effects of depot injections are irreversible and continue for some time, it is best first to try a small test dose of the preparation to be used to check for any sensitivity or other adverse effects before starting at the therapeutic dose. TTFFF

If it is decided not to admit her to hospital (if she agrees to take medications and the psychiatrist considers that she is likely to comply), it is important to arrange regular follow-up by a community psychiatric nurse and also further support from Social Services. Also, she has not yet had a physical examination. This is important to exclude organic factors in the development of her disorder, particularly in someone of her age.

Clinical Case 9

Patient 9

Mrs Maureen M, a 25-year-old married shorthand typist, presents to her general practitioner complaining that she is afraid of going out and also of using lifts. She has always been rather timid but these problems appear to be getting worse over the last three years, since an uncle to whom she was very close died suddenly of a myocardial infarct. She is seeking help now because she has recently changed jobs and her new job involves a much longer journey to work by public transport than she previously had and also she has to use lifts regularly at work and finds her fear of them a considerable handicap. Although her new office is friendly, she says that she tries to avoid conversation with her colleagues, because she is concerned about appearing foolish or gauche.

In the interview, Mrs M comes across as rather shy and awkward, and seems reluctant to be drawn into talking about the details of her problems. However, she asks directly what is wrong with her, adding that a friend with similar problems benefited considerably from some pills she was given. She asks if she too could have some medication to help her.

The general practitioner should:

A. suggest a therapeutic trial of medication (either a tricyclic antidepressant or a benzodiazepine)
B. take her blood pressure then tell her that some investigations will be arranged
C. ask for more details of the friend's complaints
D. tell her that she has agoraphobia
E. raise the possibility of a behavioural programme
F. raise the possibility of some other type of psychotherapy

The presenting problems are not yet clear—suggesting a diagnosis or outlining different treatment possibilities would be premature. The friend's illness is a red herring—Mrs M's treatment must be decided on the basis of her problems, not the friend's. It may be necessary to make this point explicitly to Mrs M. FFFFFF

It proves difficult to build up a clear picture of Maureen's symptoms, and the general practitioner has to elicit further details with a series of direct questions. Mrs M admits that she cannot use the underground at all. She sometimes manages to use buses, but not always. She will not join a bus queue if there are a number of people waiting there already, preferring under these circumstances to walk to the next stop. She finds it difficult to get into a bus if it is crowded, and prefers to find a seat as far from the door as possible, thinking that someone else is less likely to sit next to her there. On further questioning, she adds that her main concern is that, if someone sitting next to her tries to strike up a conversation with her, she would not know what to say and might make a fool of herself. She admits that she is particularly concerned that she will blush or 'clam up'. She cannot use buses during rush hours. Fortunately, her hours of work are flexible so she does not have to travel during the rush hour routinely and when this is necessary, she insists that her husband accompany her. She finds that by engrossing herself in conversation with him, she is less concerned about travelling by bus. To help her in this way, her husband has had to take the odd hour off work. Mrs M adds that fortunately, her husband's employer is very understanding. Regarding lifts, she says that she cannot get into a lift if it is already crowded. If she is in a lift and there are people standing in front of her when the doors open at her stop, she would rather stay in the lift than ask to be allowed past. She has little difficulty travelling in a lift when there is nobody else in it. As an afterthought she adds that she and her husband used to visit their local pub regularly, but now she finds this impossible and her social contacts are largely confined to her family and close friends. She also admits to difficulty shopping—she drives some distance to a supermarket to avoid using the local shops, which she found adequate for her needs in the past. She prefers not to leave the house during the day unless she has to, but often takes her dog for walks in the evening, when there are likely to be fewer people about.

On the information so far, possible diagnoses include:

A. agoraphobia
B. claustrophobia (because of her fear of lifts)
C. social phobia
D. depression
E. obsessive-compulsive disorder

She is clearly phobic. Some of her symptoms are common features of agoraphobia, like her fears of travelling by public transport or of shopping, and her need to be accompanied by her husband. In agoraphobia, key features are a reluctance to leave familiar surroundings (like home) and the fear of panicking in a situation where escape is difficult (lifts, buses, shops, and so on). However, looking at her story more carefully, her main concern is not that she will panic and thus humiliate herself, but rather that she will make a fool of herself if she has to talk to someone else. Having her husband with her means that he can do all the talking where necessary. This—the fear of situations in which one is exposed to the scrutiny of other people—is the cardinal feature of social phobia. People who are agoraphobic tend, on buses, to choose seats as close as possible to the exit, so that a quick 'escape' is possible if necessary. Also, agoraphobic people usually find more difficulty shopping in a supermarket (which is often difficult to leave in a hurry) than in small neighbourhood shops, with which they are usually familiar and in which they thus feel more confident.

Having difficulty travelling in lifts with others could be a feature of either agoraphobia or social phobia, and further questions are necessary to decide which is more likely. In Mrs M's case, her fear of lifts is having to ask others in front of her to allow her through—again consistent with social phobia. In claustrophobia, being in a lift unaccompanied is usually much worse than using the lift when there are others in it. Any phobia may be secondary to depression, and Mrs M must be asked about the features of depression, but there is nothing in the history so far to indicate that she is depressed. Some people who become phobic try to cope with their anxiety by taking more alcohol—it is important to ask about this also. There is nothing in the history to suggest that this might be obsessive-compulsive disorder (although obsessional trends have been noted to accompany agoraphobia). TFTTF

Clinical Case 9

She denies any symptoms of depression or any increase in her consumption of alcohol beyond the level of 'social drinking', adding that although she and her husband used to go to the pub together regularly, they seldom do so now because she finds this too uncomfortable, admits that when she becomes anxious, she feels sweaty and thinks that she blushes. She cannot help feeling that others notice how uncomfortable she looks. When anxious also, she gets a strange feeling as though she is outside herself, looking at herself being uncomfortable. This sensation worries her greatly—she admits that, when the sensation comes, it sometimes occurs to her that she must be losing her mind. This sensation she describes:

A. makes the diagnosis of social phobia less likely
B. is a phenomenon indicative of psychosis
C. indicates that her problem is particularly severe
D. may occur in the absence of any psychiatric disorder
E. is derealisation

She is describing depersonalisation. This is a common accompaniment of anxiety, even in people who cannot be considered psychiatrically ill. This has no bearing on the severity of her phobic problems. FFFTF

The general practitioner adopts a working diagnosis of social phobia, possibly with features of agoraphobia. At this stage, appropriate treatment options include:

A. prescribing a two-week course of diazepam 2 mg to be taken up to three times daily before going in journeys by public transport
B. prescribing amitriptyline 25 mg b.d. in preference to a benzodiazepine to avoid serious problems with dependence
C. giving her (or suggest she gets) an audiotape of relaxation exercises
D. referral for behaviour therapy
E. referral for exploratory psychotherapy
F. referral for cognitive therapy
G. involving Mrs M's husband in the treatment

It is very unlikely that a two-week course of diazepam would eliminate Mrs M's difficulties. Even if she became less anxious on diazepam, her symptoms are likely to return when the diazepam is discontinued. Although the sedative effects of amitriptyline might help Mrs M's anxiety, no evidence was found for depression and prescription of amitriptyline is therefore not indicated. Mrs M's problems began shortly after the sudden and unexpected death of her uncle. The relationship of this event to her symptoms, together with other possible underlying causes of her present difficulties, could be pursued in exploratory psychotherapy. However, this is inevitably a slow process and she has presented at this time because she is becoming increasingly handicapped by her symptoms (at work, for example). Thus exploratory psychotherapy is worth considering, but not at this stage, when Mrs M really wants symptomatic relief. This could be provided by behaviour therapy or by cognitive therapy. Relaxation management is commonly acknowledged as a useful component of either of these approaches, although some experts have questioned its efficacy. Mrs M's husband has clearly become involved in managing her symptoms and it would be appropriate to involve him in her treatment plan. FFTTFTT

It is not necessary to refer the patient for specialist help. Depending on his own training, the general practitioner might offer a course of treatment himself. In this instance, he decides to offer Mrs M a brief course of behaviour therapy. He gives her a tape on relaxation techniques to listen to and they agree a further appointment. Which of the following 'homework' tasks would be appropriate for Mrs M to complete before the next visit?

A. recording her level of anxiety in different situations on a scale of 0 (no anxiety) to 10 (the worst anxiety she has ever experienced)
B. writing a list of reasons why her uncle's death might have precipitated her symptoms
C. leaving her house a specified number of times each day
D. making at least one bus journey without her husband in the rush hour
E. keeping a diary of her activities (at 2–3 hourly intervals) and noting beside each one how anxious it made her feel

'Homework' is an important component of behavioural and also cognitive approaches, allowing the therapeutic work to continue outside the sessions with the therapist. The main objective in treatment is alleviating Mrs M's anxiety about being in the company of others. The homework task must be relevant to this aim and, more particularly, directly related to Mrs M's symptoms. The task must also be explicitly defined and not so difficult that Mrs M is unlikely to achieve it. Keeping a record of her activities and quantifying how anxious she becomes while performing them provide important 'baseline' information about the extent of her problem and her present level of functioning. Information from this diary might also help to construct a hierarchy of feared situations for a systematic desensitisation programme. It is not clear from the information thus far that going outdoors is itself a problem, or that the frequency of Mrs M's going outdoors relates to her phobia. Thus this task is not sufficiently specific. Focusing on her uncle's death might reveal something about the underlying causes of her phobia, but is not directly related to the symptoms themselves. From her account, making an unaccompanied bus journey in the rush hour is likely to be too difficult at this stage, and, if set as a homework task, may discourage Mrs M from continuing with the therapy. TFFFT

Mrs M returns the following week, without any diary. She says that she has been too busy to keep any record of her activities. She again asks for medication. The doctor should now:

A. tell Mrs M that she requires specialist help and refer her to a psychiatrist
B. suggest that Mrs M try again to record her activities and her anxiety and give her another appointment

C. accept that she is likely to be too busy to do much homework between sessions

D. help her, during the interview, to fill out her diary for the previous one or two days

E. explain again the aims and method of the treatment, even though this uses up valuable time in the session

F. conclude that Mrs M is unsuitable for behaviour therapy

There are numerous reasons why patients fail to do their homework assignments. These include not understanding what the treatment programme (or homework task) is about, seeing the task as too difficult (or too trivial) and fearing that focusing more on their symptoms is likely to make them feel worse rather than better. Given how concerned Mrs M is about her problems and their impact on her life, it seems hard to accept that lack of time would have prevented her from completing the diary. It would be unnecessary and unfortunate if the doctor gave up at this stage. However, merely asking her to try again to do the same task for another week is unlikely to succeed. The doctor should make sure Mrs M understands the treatment programme. It is often helpful to fill in one or two days' activities with the patient, to demonstrate what is required. Even if she ultimately fails to keep her diary of activities, this is not absolutely essential and another behavioural programme could be considered. FFFTTF

Further discussion reveals that Mrs M is concerned that colleagues at work might see her filling in the diary and catch a glimpse of what she had written. She would be very embarrassed if this happened. Mrs M discusses possible ways of overcoming this problem with the doctor. She could record each day's activities as accurately as possible at home every evening. She decides on a more creative solution—she speaks and writes fluent Spanish (her husband is from Spain) and decides to keep her diary in Spanish.

She comes to her next appointment with her diary, which she has succeeded in filling out, and translates her records for the doctor. Her records confirm that she becomes most anxious in situations in which she might have to interact with strangers. Mrs M and the doctor agree to tackle the problem with the lifts at work first. Work on this might include:

A. rehearsing or role-playing what she would say to someone blocking her way to the lift door when she wanted to get out from the lift

B. setting her the task of travelling in the lift at work a given number of times each day, recording how anxious she felt on each occasion

C. getting her in the interview to imagine stepping into a crowded lift and then encouraging her to make use of the relaxation exercises to try to reduce her anxiety

D. recording how frequently she is able to travel to work by bus

E. getting her to imagine how anxious she would feel if the lift in which she was travelling stopped between floors

Details of her bus journeys are not directly relevant to the problem with lifts, except in that they are both related to her fear of associating with strangers. She has not so far expressed a particular fear of being stuck in a lift—there is thus no advantage to choose this as a homework task. It is important to keep the treatment as clearly focused as possible. The other options are all appropriate. In the sessions, Mrs M can learn how to use her relaxation exercises to diminish her anxiety, and also practice what to say and do when she wants to step past someone in the lift. Practising travelling in the lift is also important. This can be graded, starting at a level Mrs M is likely to achieve. For example, she might begin by using the lift at least twice when she is at work, except during the lunch hour when the lift is invariably full. As her anxiety reduces and she becomes more confident, the number of journeys is increased, and one journey is included which must be made during the lunch hour. TTTFF

Initially, Mrs M records anxiety levels of 7 or 8 on each occasion she steps into a lift. After four weeks, she rates her anxiety on most occasions in the lift at 2–3, but still records anxiety levels of 5 on her lunchtime journeys. She no longer avoids using the lift, and feels confident that she will continue to feel better with further practice. At this stage:

A. it is unlikely that she will have any further episodes of considerable anxiety in a lift in the following few weeks
B. the treatment may have had some impact on her other symptoms
C. it is necessary to continue working on the same problem (using lifts) until she experiences no anxiety for the treatment to be effective
D. the chances of a relapse would be reduced if Mrs M had some exploratory psychotherapy to discover more about the underlying cause of her symptoms
E. it may now be necessary to start a behavioural programme aimed at reducing her fear of travelling by bus

Occasional 'relapses' do occur after treatment of conditions like phobias—patients should be warned to expect them and also be reassured that a recurrence of any of their symptoms does not necessarily mean that they will forfeit their progress and return to their previous anxious state. In the case of problems like Mrs M's, it is quite likely that tackling one problem or symptom produces benefits for others. For example, acquiring more skill and confidence in addressing strangers in lifts is likely to make it easier for Mrs M to face a similar prospect when travelling by bus. However, it may be necessary to tackle the different problems separately. In Mrs M's case, if her difficulties in using buses need to be addressed in a behavioural programme, it would be helpful to involve her husband, if possible. There is no necessity to remove the symptoms completely for the behaviour therapy to succeed—the point at which a particular piece of work is considered complete can be agreed by the therapist and patient together. For phobias and other problems treated symptomatically using behaviour therapy, there is no convincing evidence to date that addressing the underlying cause(s) of the problem decreases the chance of relapse. FTFFT

Clinical Case 10

Patient 10

Joseph K, a 74-year-old ex-accountant, presents to his general practitioner complaining of 'pains in the head'. It proves very difficult to elicit precise details of these pains, beyond Mr K's observation that they are 'shooting' pains, sometimes behind both eyes, and sometimes across the top of his head from forehead to neck. He also complains of pains in his neck. He denies any respite from these pains while he is awake—he feels pain the moment he awakes, and the pains are with him until he falls asleep. Asked whether the pain prevents him from falling asleep, he is at first uncertain, then answers that, usually, he has little trouble falling asleep, although he awakes much earlier than is usual for him. On direct questioning, he is unsure whether or not he wakes so early because of pain. He knows of nothing that will ease his pains. He has tried a variety of analgesics (that he has bought himself and also prescribed by his general practitioner) with no effect whatsoever. Initially, he denies that anything specific makes the pains worse. On further questioning, it emerges that his pains began about nine months ago, shortly after the death of his wife. He has had the pains since that time and now admits that they become much worse sometimes when he thinks of his wife. As he talks about his wife, he is close to tears, but does not cry. He remembers that he was completely free of the pains for a few days, when he went to stay with his only granddaughter, with whom he has always enjoyed a close relationship. She has recently been married and is shortly to emigrate overseas with her husband. On direct questioning, he admits to feeling very low in his spirits, but asks the doctor whether he too would not feel so miserable if he had to endure such pains. He used to enjoy meeting friends, gardening and painting but he has now stopped all of these activities—he says his pains prevent him from concentrating on them.

Mr K has already been fully investigated for his head pains by the neurologists. Thorough physical examinations and a battery of tests (including an EEG) have proven negative. He was also prescribed amitriptyline, but stopped taking this after three days because he found the side-effects intolerable.

Despite reassurance from both his general practitioner and the neurologist, Mr K is convinced that there is something seriously wrong and suspects that he has a brain tumour. He returns to his general practitioner, saying that he wishes to have a CAT brain scan.

On the information so far given:

A. the observation that Mr K's pains get much worse sometimes when he thinks about his dead wife indicates that the pains are of 'psychological' rather than organic origin

B. if enough details can be elicited about the pains, the properties of the pains will allow one to decide accurately whether or not they have an organic origin

C. the clinical picture is consistent with the diagnosis of an atypical (masked) depression

D. the doctor should tell Mr K that he (the doctor) is very confident that there is nothing seriously wrong with Mr K, to reassure him

E. the doctor should make it clear to Mr K that his pains have a psychological rather than a physical cause and recommend referral to a psychiatrist

The history obtained from Mr K suggests that there may be an important emotional component to his symptoms. It may be more than coincidental that the pains began after his wife's death, and that they become worse when he thinks of her. Also, he felt considerably better for a brief period when he was with his granddaughter (who is also now 'leaving' him, to get married and to emigrate). In addition, he admits to some features of depression. He feels low in his spirits, has given up activities he used to enjoy and also has early morning wakening. These features are certainly consistent with his having an atypical (or masked) depression.

It is unwise to exclude an organic cause contributing to his pains on the basis of the history alone. This may be possible in some extreme cases, where it is evident from the patient's account that his symptoms cannot be adequately explained in terms of physiological and anatomical principles. More commonly, however, emotional factors will affect the intensity of the pain, as well as the patient's perception of its nature and properties. This happens whatever the aetiology of the pain. Thus the observation that Mr K's pains change when he thinks about his wife or when he is with his granddaughter does not exclude an organic component to the pains.

Even though it is not possible confidently to exclude an organic cause for the pains, the doctor must form some judgement about the relative contributions of organic and emotional factors in each case, remembering that these two groups of factors are not mutually exclusive and both need to be addressed in assessment and treatment. In Mr K's case, he has already been investigated but has not been reassured that his pains are not due to a brain tumour. It is thus appropriate at this stage to try to examine the emotional factors contributing to his pain. However, reassuring Mr K that there is nothing seriously wrong is likely to antagonise him—for him, his pains are very distressing, and there *is* something wrong. Many people find it difficult to comprehend that pain, especially when it is severe, can present without a physical cause. Mr K's request for a CAT brain scan makes his attitude clear. Offering him a psychiatric assessment on the basis that his pain is clearly 'psychological', without further discussion, is adding insult to injury. Psychiatric referral must be carefully negotiated with the patient, even if the doctor feels convinced that this is the appropriate step. FFTFF

The general practitioner explains to Mr K that pain often has an emotional component, whatever its cause. Mr K reluctantly agrees that this may be worth pursuing and eventually accepts referral to a psychiatrist who is particularly interested and experienced in treating the emotional aspects of pain. In the first psychiatric interview, it emerges that his wife died from cancer of the colon. She had been ill for only a few months before her death, but had borne her suffering very bravely, until shortly before she died, when she became very tearful and anxious. He describes their 51-year marriage as 'perfect', and has difficulty in keeping back the tears when talking about her. He adds that they always did everything together and he finds it impossible to do anything at all now that she is not longer alive.

Mr K is reluctant to consider taking more medications which might give him

Clinical Case 10

further side-effects, and the psychiatrist decides to use a psychotherapeutic approach, along cognitive-behavioural lines (cognitive therapy often includes behavioural components—see MCQ 134). The psychiatrist explains something about the cognitive approach and how the therapy sessions will be structured, and he and Mr K agree to meet regularly for five sessions before reviewing progress. Which of the following would be appropriate for a cognitive approach in this case?

A. asking Mr K in the interview to rate how severe his pains are then to think about the loss of his wife before rating his pains again
B. suggesting that he keeps a diary of his weekly actitivities and at the same time rate the severity of his pains
C. avoiding any mention of his pains in the therapy sessions, to concentrate more on his symptoms of depression
D. asking Mr K to write down a list of reasons why he believes that his pains must be due to a brain tumour

Cognitive therapy emphasises the links between beliefs and emotions, and aims to get the patient to discover how these links operate and to exert control over them. It may be possible to arrange a 'contract' with Mr K such that he and the psychiatrist explore his bereavement quite separately from his pains. However, pain is Mr K's main symptom and his chief concern, thus avoiding all mention of it is likely to antagonise him.

Getting Mr K to list the evidence in favour of his pain being due to a brain tumour is likely to yield more information about his assumptions and beliefs regarding his symptoms. He has already mentioned that he is unable to do anything because of his pain—this may be more a belief than a fact, and can be tested out by getting him to complete a daily diary of his activities. The best way to demonstrate a link between Mr K's pains and his emotions is to show such a link during the interview itself. Thinking about his wife is likely (from his own account) to make the pain worse. Thus it might be helpful in better understanding his symptoms to get him to rate his pain (on a 0–10 scale, with 0 being no pain, 10 the worst pain he has ever had) before and after he has 'provoked' his symptoms by thinking of his wife. TTFT

Mr K is very reluctant to see how, in the interview, thinking about his wife changes his pains. After further discussion of the possible links between thoughts and emotions, the psychiatrist and Mr K agree that, as a 'homework' task, Mr K will compile a list of the evidence for and against his pain being due to a brain tumour. He is also to keep a daily record of his activities.

Mr K returns the following week to his next appointment, having failed to make out his list. He has, however, managed to keep an activity diary, which is virtually empty, apart from references to mundane housekeeping tasks and occasionally watching television. Mr K asserts that there is no point in doing anything more than this, as he is bound to fail and then will feel even worse. As evidence of this, he tells the psychiatrist that he tried to paint his granddaughter's portrait from memory but found himself unable to get into the work. He again raises the possibility of a brain scan.

The psychiatrist should now:

A. conclude that a cognitive approach is unlikely to work and try to persuade Mr K to reconsider taking an antidepressant
B. move away from considering Mr K's daily activities and concentrate instead on his pains
C. attempt to confront Mr K with his (the psychiatrist's) view that Mr K's pains have a largely psychological basis
D. suggest, in order to improve Mr K's compliance with the treatment, that he would arrange a CT brain scan
E. probe further Mr K's assertion that he is bound to fail at anything he tries

Psychotherapy does not entail one approach that is 'right' and others that are 'wrong'—a particular problem can usually be tackled in more than one way. If one specific direction of work does not succeed, it may be appropriate to consider another. It would certainly be premature to abandon the cognitive approach altogether on the basis of Mr K's homework. Furthermore, Mr K has brought additional evidence about his perceived inability to do anything, which is worth exploring in more detail. To shift completely to examine his pain further would be to neglect this evidence. Until Mr K himself is ready to see that his pains have a psychological origin (having demonstrated this to himself), confronting him with the psychiatrist's views would be unhelpful. Using the CAT scan as a form of 'bribe' would not be helpful in the long run. FFFFT

Mr K and the psychiatrist discuss his failure to paint his granddaughter's portrait. Mr K admits that this is a very ambitious project and that he has tried in the past to paint from memory but never been satisfied with the results. The psychiatrist suggests that Mr K is at present thinking of 'all-or-nothing' terms, extrapolating from his failure at an acknowledged difficult task to everything else he does. He points out that such 'all-or-nothing' thinking is common when people feel low, as is the assumption, which Mr K also appears to have, that nothing can be done to change things. It appears that Mr K has the automatic thought 'No matter what I do, I am bound to fail.' Further discussion allows Mr K and the psychiatrist to formulate another possible belief—'There is no way that I can get pleasure or enjoyment from anything without my wife being there too.'

Appropriate homework tasks to follow on from this session would be:

A. getting Mr K to attempt less ambitious activities which he used to enjoy and to rate each for the pleasure it gives him on a 0–10 scale
B. getting Mr K to rate the severity of his pains at intervals during the day
C. asking him to spend at least three hours daily in his garden (which he admits has become rather overgrown)
D. getting Mr K to write down any other negative thoughts he might have

As with homework assignments in behavioural therapy (see case 9), the tasks set should be circumscribed, explicitly stated and attainable. Having identified one or possibly two **dysfunctional thoughts**, it is appropriate for the homework to focus on these. The aim here is to get Mr K to attempt previously enjoyable activities (but in a less ambitious manner than before) and test his assumptions of inevitable failure and deriving no pleasure by getting him to record, for each activity, how much pleasure and how much mastery he experiences from the activity. Setting too many tasks for one homework assignment is risky, because the patient may not achieve them and thus feel even more of a failure. However, in this case, one aim is to demonstrate for the patient the link between his pains and his emotions. Thus it would be worth asking him to record the severity of his pain along with his activity diary. Spending three hours daily at work in an overgrown garden is likely to be too ambitious a task—it would be best to let Mr K set his own pace, discouraging him from attempting anything too ambitious. Usually, negative thoughts can be 'captured' by the patient when he becomes aware that he feels miserable (or, in this case, perhaps when his pains are severe) and searches for the automatic thoughts underlying this emotional state. This is a technique to which the patient must be introduced by the therapist—it usually requires some work with patient and therapist in the therapy sessions. Simply asking Mr K to write down any negative thoughts he might have is not sufficiently specific a task and again runs a high risk of failing. TTFF

At his next therapy session, Mr K appears quite animated. He has tried to do some gardening, done a little painting and also listened to some of his jazz records for the first time in months. To his surprise, he has found that he has managed to enjoy the records and has also gained pleasure from the garden. In other words, having set himself more appropriate goals than previously, he has demonstrated to himself that he can still experience enjoyment and mastery, which he now accepts as evidence against the belief that he is bound always to fail. He now finds himself better able to sleep than previously, and is also eating more. Unfortunately, he has not recorded the severity of his pains, but says that the pains have been as bad as ever and were not significantly influenced by his activities. The psychiatrist reviews with Mr K how his previous beliefs appeared to 'trap' him, setting up what became a self-fulfilling prophesy. Mr K concedes that the same could possibly be true regarding his pain and agrees to try again to monitor its severity. He returns the following week having succeeded in monitoring his pains. Reviewing his recordings, he and the psychiatrist agree that his pains are consistently affected by his mood (note that, although he already knows that his pain became worse when he thought about his wife, he has now demonstrated to himself not only that his pain symptoms are more intimately linked with his emotions than he had previously considered possible, but also that he can to some extent control his emotions and hence also the pains).

Over the next few weeks, he continues to make progress. Having rated his pains at 7–8/10 on most days previously, the pain ratings are now commonly 2 or 3. Having reviewed the evidence for and against his pains being due to a brain tumour, he is now prepared to accept that there are other explanations for such severe pain, having demonstrated how it is affected by his emotions. He no longer has the features of depression with which he presented and is very active in his garden and with his hobbies. He continues to be very reluctant to think or talk too much about his wife in the therapy sessions. Looking into this further, he and the psychiatrist agree that another of his beliefs is likely to be, 'If I show too much of my feelings, I shall (somehow) fall apart.' Mr K admits that he suspects this happened to his wife. She had always been rather a stoical woman, but died shortly after she had allowed her feelings of distress out into the open. However, overall, Mr K feels much better and believes he can get back to a lifestyle with which he can be comfortable.

At this point:

A. it is vital to pursue his reluctance to show his feelings
B. unless his unresolved feelings about his wife are addressed, he will inevitably relapse
C. he should be recommended to have exploratory psychotherapy
D. it is vital to pursue Mr K's belief that if he shows his feelings, he'll fall apart
E. the psychiatrist should now persuade Mr K to accept a trial of antidepressants

Mr K's difficulties have not entirely resolved—he still admits to a little pain and refuses to talk about his wife. However, at this stage it is not clear that he wants any further help. He appears quite happy with his progress, and has on several occasions demonstrated his reluctance to 'expose' his feelings. It is not necessary to address this problem—as with any other form of therapy, likely benefit must be balanced against potential cost. Exploratory psychotherapy would certainly necessitate his confronting his feelings, and would thus be inappropriate at this stage, given his attitude. He has lost the symptoms of depression he had previously, and there is therefore no indication for antidepressants. FFFFF

It may well be that these unresolved problems will cause Mr K distress in the future, although there is no satisfactory way of predicting this. In finishing the therapy, the psychiatrist warns Mr K of this possibility and suggests that Mr K ask his general practitioner to refer him back to the psychiatric clinic should the pains become worse or Mr K again becomes depressed.

Appendix

For multiple choice questions to be an adequate test of knowledge, it is helpful for the student to know how others score on the same questions and how well the questions themselves discriminate between better and poorer students. The questions listed below have all been tested on medical students who have completed a two-month attachment in psychiatry. Each question was tested on

MCQ number	Mean score	r	MCQ number	Mean score	r	MCQ number	Mean score	r
2	2.0	.15	49	−.7	.22	95	1.3	.47
3	2.1	.16	50	2.5	.51	96	1.9	−.07
5	1.2	.53	51	1.6	.19	97	1.2	.28
6	3.6	−.15	53	2.1	.01	98	2.0	.55
7	2.0	.31	54	3.5	.27	100	1.6	.14
8	2.9	.13	55	1.8	.41	101	1.1	.35
9	2.5	.24	56	2.1	.31	103	1.8	−.34
11	.9	.19	59	2.0	.21	104	2.1	.48
12	3.6	.46	60	.8	.24	107	2.2	.39
14	3.7	.49	61	3.8	.36	109	1.7	.43
16	1.9	.58	62	4.5	.09	110	1.2	.15
17	2.3	.12	63	2.1	.57	111	1.9	.35
18	2.4	.20	64	−.5	.39	112	1.6	.34
19	2.1	−.24	65	−.2	.51	113	2.1	.31
20	1.8	.15	67	2.7	.47	114	1.3	0
22	1.2	.10	69	2.3	.06	115	1.7	.17
23	.5	.64	70	.8	.29	116	1.0	.25
25	−.7	.18	73	1.3	.09	118	3.0	.04
27	3.6	.23	74	3.1	.45	119	1.7	.38
28	4.5	.04	75	1.5	.11	120	1.8	.30
29	1.6	.41	77	−1.1	.17	121	1.2	.30
31	1.9	.11	79	.1	.33	122	1.6	−.02
33	4.1	.01	80	.9	.37	123	1.3	−.13
34	1.9	.49	81	3.1	.18	124	0.0	.25
35	2.1	.23	82	2.6	.29	125	−.7	.34
38	3.4	.11	84	.4	.30	126	.9	.37
39	.8	.06	85	2.1	.61	127	2.8	.32
40	3.9	.46	86	2.0	.40	128	3.4	.38
41	1.6	.32	87	3.8	.22	129	1.6	.43
43	1.7	.14	89	1.8	.18	130	1.5	.43
44	2.8	.40	90	.8	.38	133	3.2	.30
46	.9	.16	92	1.8	.10	134	2.3	.18
47	4.3	.05	93	2.5	.23	135	2.4	.07
48	1.7	.30						

25–35 students. The easier questions tend to have higher mean scores (range −5 to +5). In addition to the means, the correlation is given between the students' scores on a particular question and their overall score on a 50-question MCQ examination. Questions which are good at discriminating between better and poorer students have higher values of r, the correlation coefficient. One reason why r may be low is that the question is ambiguous. However, we have tried as far as possible to eliminate such questions and there are a number of other reasons why r might remain low; for example, strong and weak candidates may score equally well on a relatively easy question.

Subject Index

Throughout the text the symbol ★ identifies topics that are covered in more than one MCQ.

Aetiology   17, 19
Affective disorder
  bipolar   71, 81
  unipolar   71
Affective disorders
  aetiology   77
  epidemiology   76
  treatment   78, 79, 80, 168, 207–209
Agoraphobia   93, 94
Akathisia   187
Alcohol dependence   110
Alcoholic blackouts   114
Alcoholic dementia   114, 212, 214
Alcoholic hallucinosis   113
Alcoholism   110
  detection   115
  epidemiology   111
Alzheimer-type dementia, see Dementia,
  Alzheimer-type
Amnesia
  post-traumatic   42
  transient global   23
Anhedonia   69, 169
Anorexia nervosa   124, 127, 223–227
Anticholinergic drugs   187, 191
Antidepressants   79, 165, 168, 180, 182
Antipsychotic drugs   61, 62, 185, 186,
  187, 189, 217
Antisocial personality disorder, see
  Personality disorder, psychopathic
Anxiety   91, 165, 166, 168
  phobic, see Phobias
Attachment   147
Attention, see Cognitive examination

Baby blues   174
Behaviour therapy   139, 198, 201, 235,
  245
Benzodiazepines   184
Brain syndromes
  acute   22, 25–27, 211, 228
  assessment   44, 228
  chronic, see Dementia

Briquet's syndrome   97
Bulimia nervosa   126, 127

Cannabis   120
Care order   152
Cheese reaction   180, 182
Child abuse   107, 151
Classification (of psychiatric disorders)   4
Cognitions   82, 200
Cognitive examination   12, 13, 22, 44,
  231
Cognitive impairment   22, 25
Cognitive therapy   78, 82, 200, 250–253
Compulsions   6, 96
Concentration, see Cognitive examination
Conduct disorders (in children)   146, 150
Confabulation   23
Confusional states, acute, see Brain
  syndromes, acute
Coping   158, 177
Countertransference   193
Cultural differences   15, 16, 111, 130,
  170, 172

Defence mechanisms   177, 193
Deliberate self-harm   113, 133, 134,
  207, 218–222
Delinquency   150
Delirium   26
Delirium tremens   26, 110, 113, 114,
  212, 229
Delusions   9, 57
  in affective disorder   72
  in schizophrenia   57
Dementia   28, 30, 31, 32, 230
  Alzheimer-type   30
  management   34
  multi-infarct   31
  reversible causes   32
Denial   177
Dependence, drug   117, 184
Depersonalisation   75, 100, 244

Depression
  biological symptoms   68, 69, 70
  classification   70
  endogenous, see Melancholia
  in medical inpatients   166, 168, 177
  masked   71, 168, 248
  neurotic   69, 70, 75
  postnatal   174
  psychotic   68, 70, 72, 209
  'resistant'   79, 181
Derealisation   100
Desensitisation, systematic   93, 198
Disorientation, see Cognitive examination
Drug abuse   117
Drug dependence, see Dependence, drug
DSM-IIIR   3
Dyskinesia, tardive, see Tardive
  dyskinesia
Dystonia, acute   187

ECT, see Electroconvulsive therapy
Ejaculation
  premature   137, 140, 233
  retarded   137
  retrograde   141
Electroconvulsive therapy   61, 78, 79,
  80, 174, 192, 209
Electroencephalography   40, 41, 44
Emotional disorders (in children)   146
Enuresis   146, 149
Epidemiology, general   15, 164
Epilepsy   38, 39, 41
  temporal lobe   39
Erectile dysfunction   138, 139, 233
Exhibitionism   113, 142
Expressed emotion   60, 62, 217
Extrapyramidal symptoms   187, 191

Fetishism   142
First rank symptoms   8, 10, 48, 54, 216
Forgetfulness, senescent   36
Formal thought disorder   8
Frontal lobe syndrome   42
Fugue state   100
Functional psychosis, see Psychosis

General hospital psychiatry, see Liaison
  psychiatry
Genetics   17
Grief reactions   84, 85

Hallucinations   11
  in depression   72
  in schizophrenia   57
Head injury   42
Hydrocephalus, normal pressure   32

Hyperventilation   175
Hypochondriasis   84, 101, 172
Hysteria   97
Hysterical amnesia   100
Hysterical conversion   97, 98, 172
Hysterical dissociation   97, 100

ICD-9   3
Idea, overvalued   6
Idea of reference   6
Illness behaviour, abnormal   101
Illusions   11
Incest   151
Insight
  in psychotherapy   196
  lack of   4, 11
Intellectual retardation   153

Jealousy, morbid, see Morbid jealousy

Korsakoff's psychosis   23, 114, 212

Liaison psychiatry   156, 166
Life events   19, 60, 77, 160
Lithium   78, 81, 183

Malingering   97, 172
Mania   73, 74
Manic-depressive disorder, see Affective
  disorder, bipolar
Melancholia   69, 70, 169, 207
Memory   13, 23
Mental Health Act   153, 192, 202–204,
  209, 220, 238, 240
Mental state examination   6, 12
Mental subnormality   153
Models of mental illness   2
Morbid jealousy   9, 113
Mourning, guided   86
Multiple personality   100
Munchausen's syndrome   107

Neuroleptic drugs, see Antipsychotic
  drugs
Neuroleptic malignant syndrome   190
Neuroses
  aetiology   89
  epidemiology   88
  outcome   90
  undifferentiated   88
Neurosis   4, 88
Neurosyphilis   32

Obsessions   6, 96
Obsessive-compulsive neurosis   96, 198
Opiates, dependence on   118

Organic psychosis, *see* Psychosis
Organic reaction, acute, *see* Brain
    syndromes, acute

Paedophilia 142
Pain 170, 248
Panic attacks 91, 175
Paraphrenia 36, 237–239
Parasuicide, *see* Deliberate self-harm
Parkinsonism, drug-induced 187
Passivity phenomena 54
Perseveration 28
Personality disorder 5, 104, 106, 107
    psychopathic 106
Phenomenology 3
    school, *see* School refusal
    social 93, 95, 243
Phobias 75, 91, 93, 243
Pick's disease 32
Place of Safety Order 152
Post-traumatic syndrome 42
Postnatal psychosis, *see* Psychosis,
    postnatal
Pressure of speech 8, 73
Primary care, psychiatric morbidity in
    164, 165
Pseudodementia, depressive 24, 32, 36
Pseudohallucinations 11
Psychogenic pain disorder 170
Psychopathy, *see* Personality disorder,
    psychopathic
Psychosis 4
    postnatal 174
Psychosomatic disorders 15, 158
Psychosomatic medicine 156
Psychosomatics 157
Psychotherapy 193, 194–201
    behavioural, *see* Behaviour therapy
    brief focal 196
    cognitive, *see* Cognitive therapy
    exploratory 195, 196, 197, 199, 201
    supportive 196
Puerperal depression, *see* Depression,
    postnatal
Puerperal psychosis, *see* Psychosis
    postnatal

Reading retardation 147
Reality orientation 35

Schizophrenia
    aetiology 51, 52
    classification 55

epidemiology 50
first rank symptoms, *see* First rank
    symptoms
management 61, 62, 64
negative symptoms 56
neuropathology 53, 59
positive symptoms 55
prognosis 52, 55, 59, 60
Schizophreniform psychosis 18, 48
School refusal 148
Seizures
    epileptic, *see* Epilepsy
    pseudoepileptic 40, 41
Sexual deviance 142
Sexual dysfunction, treatment 139,
    234–236
Sexual response 136
Solvent abuse 121
Somatisation 16
Somatisation disorder 172
Stress 158, 160
Stupor 26
Suicidal intent 134, 208, 220
Suicide 130, 131
    attempted, *see* Deliberate self-harm
Suicide risk 132
Systematic desensitisation, *see*
    Desensitisation, systematic

Tardive dyskinesia 37, 59, 186, 189
Terminal illness 177
Thought alienation 8, 54
Thought broadcast, *see* Thought
    alienation
Thought echo 54
Thought insertion, *see* Thought alienation
Thought withdrawal, *see* Thought
    alienation
Transference 193
Transsexualism 142
Transvestism 142
Tricyclic antidepressants, *see*
    Antidepressants
    overdose 208, 218
Truancy 148
Type A behaviour 162

Unconscious mechanisms 193

Vaginismus 137, 139

Wernicke's encephalopathy 26, 114,
    229